The Virtuous Psychiatrist

International Perspectives in Philosophy and Psychiatry

Series editors
KWM (Bill) Fulford, Katherine Morris, John Z Sadler,
and Giovanni Stanghellini

Volumes in the series

The Virtuous Psychiatrist

Character Ethics in Psychiatric Practice

Jennifer Radden

John Z. Sadler

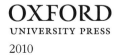

OXFORD
UNIVERSITY PRESS
2010

OXFORD
UNIVERSITY PRESS

Oxford University Press, Inc., publishes works that further
Oxford University's objective of excellence
in research, scholarship, and education.

Oxford New York
Auckland Cape Town Dar es Salaam Hong Kong Karachi
Kuala Lumpur Madrid Melbourne Mexico City Nairobi
New Delhi Shanghai Taipei Toronto

With offices in
Argentina Austria Brazil Chile Czech Republic France Greece
Guatemala Hungary Italy Japan Poland Portugal Singapore
South Korea Switzerland Thailand Turkey Ukraine Vietnam

Copyright © 2010 by Oxford University Press, Inc.

Published by Oxford University Press, Inc.
198 Madison Avenue, New York, New York 10016
www.oup.com

Oxford is a registered trademark of Oxford University Press

Library of Congress Cataloging-in-Publication Data
Radden, Jennifer.
The virtuous psychiatrist : character ethics in psychiatric practice /
Jennifer Radden, John Z. Sadler.
p. ; cm. — (International perspectives in philosophy and psychiatry)
Includes bibliographical references.
ISBN 978-0-19-538937-1
1. Psychiatric ethics. I. Sadler, John Z., 1953– II. Title.
III. Series: International perspectives in philosophy and psychiatry.
[DNLM: 1. Psychiatry—ethics. 2. Ethical Theory. 3. Professional Role.
4. Virtues. WM 62 R124v 2010]
RC455.2.E8R33 2010
174.2'9689—dc22   2009019399

9 8 7 6 5 4 3 2 1

Printed in the United States of America
on acid-free paper

For Joan M. Fordyce, who understands the art of unselfing.
Jennifer Radden

For my family, because my virtue should honor your love.
John Z. Sadler

Acknowledgments

This project was completed with support from the US Federal Government. We gratefully acknowledge grants from the National Library of Medicine (2002–2005) and the National Endowment for the Humanities (2000).

In addition, Jennifer Radden benefited from time as a visiting scholar at the Center for Human Bioethics at Monash University (1999) and as the HLA Hart visiting research fellow at Merton College, Oxford (2006).

Opportunities to try out these ideas with practitioners and moral philosophers were provided by the Ethics Board at McLean Hospital in Belmont; the departments of psychiatry at Massachusetts General Hospital in Boston (1999), and St Vincent's Hospital in Melbourne (2005); the Massachusetts Mental Health Center Law and Psychiatry Program (2005); the American Psychiatric Association Taskforce on Ethics (2001–2008), at meetings of the American Psychiatric Association (2004) and the Association for the Advancement of Philosophy and Psychiatry (2005); the New Zealand Bioethics Conference (2006); Lancaster University Philosophy Department (2006); the International Network of Philosophy and Psychiatry (2008); and the University of Pennsylvania Schools of Medicine, Social Policy, and Law, and the Strecker Psychiatric Society (2009). The advice, encouragement, and gentle direction provided by individuals in each of these settings have contributed incalculably.

Others also deserve heartfelt thanks from Jennifer Radden, including many working in moral philosophy and virtue theory; peers on the Executive Board of the Association for the Advancement of Philosophy and Psychiatry, members of PHAEDRA, colleagues at the Philosophy Department of the University of Massachusetts at Boston. Finally, thanks go to Peter Ohlin at Oxford University Press, editor without peer; Frank Keefe, unmatched critical reader; Beatrice Radden Keefe, cover design expert *extraordinaire*; and not to be forgotten, James G. Keefe.

Contents

The Virtuous Psychiatrist

Introduction

In today's vast and burgeoning literature on biomedical ethics, oriented though it so often is around case material, cases from psychiatry are few and far between. And as a separate field, psychiatric and mental health ethics have developed only haltingly during the recent decades that have seen biomedical ethics emerge as a major area of medical and humanistic study. Is this because psychiatry so exactly mirrors other medical settings that no extra attention need be paid to it? At the very least, we believe, that is a question worth exploring.

The foundations on which our work is developed are three: the conviction that ethics is important to any professional practice, including psychiatry; the notion that the settings within which psychiatry is practiced impose ethical demands on its practitioners that are distinctive enough to those settings to warrant a separate analysis; and the belief that the emphasis on character and moral psychology in a virtue theory significantly augments our understanding of the ethical demands of psychiatric practice. Each of these tenets is, of course, arguable, and we attempt to explain and support them in the pages that follow. Finally, they may represent a perspective or point of view, rather than a fully justified ethical foundation. The strength of our discussion, we believe, lies in its preparedness to give psychiatric practice its due, and in its demonstration of the value of paying attention to the character, as much as the actions, of the practitioner in psychiatry.

All medical practice is culturally embedded, but psychiatry is unusually so. Because of this, we believe, the part played by gender in psychiatry is, in its own way, almost as critical to our discussion as the tenets just outlined. Implicated in the normative presuppositions of psychiatric practice and lore, gender stands in, here, for other such categories including race, class, and ethnicity, and is given the sustained attention that, in a longer book, each of those would have received. In addition, though, gender is a factor that is today at once unremittingly controversial and, in our era of identity politics, inescapably tied to the self (or "characterization") identity that is at the heart of the therapeutic project. Gender and gender norms are for these reasons central to our discussion.

Renewed theoretical interest in a virtue or character model of ethics such as is found in Aristotle's *Nichomachean Ethics,* and in the writing of Hume and the "sentimentalist" tradition from the eighteenth century, has engendered important research during the last several decades and enriched ideas about moral psychology, virtues, and character. Included in this work have been attempts to construe professional ethics in (Aristotelian) virtue terms, and in our theoretical discussions, we draw upon and extend the role morality developed in such research, demonstrating that—and how—the ethical practice of psychiatry depends on the character of the practitioner. Indeed, the qualities allowing clinicians to be effective in helping patients (clinical skills, knowledge, and attitudes) overlap with, and are, the very qualities that make them morally good. Exemplary clinical practices are in this sense value laden, but also virtue laden.

Although the same general ethical guidelines applicable throughout biomedical ethics also fit psychiatry, we believe they are insufficient given the distinctive features of the setting in which psychiatry is practiced (the nature of psychiatric disorder, for example, and of the therapeutic enterprise). The ethical psychiatrist not only follows rules but is also a certain sort of person. Thus, as a complement to the broader biomedical ethical guidelines, we propose adding a focus on the traits of character or virtues the ethical practitioner should cultivate, including those called for by the managed care delivery system in which much of U.S. psychiatry is today practiced.

This is not a marginal addition. Although rules and principles are also important, it is our view that virtues represent the cornerstone of ethics, from which such rules and principles are ultimately derived. In addition, aspects of the psychiatry setting and the responses it calls for, as we show in what follows, seem to include several that *cannot* be governed by rules or principles. They either are "unruly" personal responses that require long cultivation and indirect habituation or are supererogatory—demands that are beyond the capability of some people. For those and related reasons, we believe only virtue ethics will allow us to formulate an adequate ethics for psychiatric practice, with the character of the virtuous psychiatrist its centerpiece.[1]

What of the practical applications of this book? Some works of ethics offer guidelines for action, or even accounts of what one must, may, and cannot do. This is not a work of that kind. At least as it is employed here, virtue ethics offers guidance as to what character traits should be cultivated, what kind of person it is good to be. Thus, it is not regulative settings but educational ones, where clinical training is taking place, that our analyses will prove most applicable. But rather than any hard and fast rules, we offer our insights into the character of the good psychiatrist as a model for emulation, and an ideal toward which trainee practitioners might be encouraged to strive. We also note some of the pedagogy associated with this kind of moral education when it is applicable to adults.

Not all philosophers have believed that virtues can be taught; it is true (Plato doubted it, for example). With Aristotle, however, we accept that virtues can be cultivated, deepened, and augmented through habituation. Easy this may not be. But by paying careful attention to the adoption and cultivation of good responses—and these will be habits of mind, as much as behavior—people can alter their characters.

As Hume and subsequent thinkers have insisted (and Aristotle arguably neglects), some of the most important virtues involve social and affective traits—empathy, for example—stemming from natural human tendencies that can be instilled with suitable moral education and good parenting during childhood and youth. Although these social and affective virtues are preconditions for our account, we accept this aspect of character development as a given. The educational context of immediate interest to us involves young adults who have (it is hoped) already received their basic moral education. And our emphasis is on Aristotle's conception of habituation, which

---

[1] Emphasis on the character of the practitioner here is not intended to diminish the importance and efforts of the other participant in the alliance—the patient. A more complete analysis of that relationship, we concede, would acknowledge other ingredients, including other moral virtues—persistence, honesty, courage, hopefulness, flexibility, and trustfulness, for instance—of the "good patient."

better fits the setting where trainees are learning the ideals and responses of their particular professional role.

This is a book about moral psychology, and the meta-ethical theory underwriting the claims we make here are not our immediate subject. Briefly though: we speak of states of affairs such as the features of the psychiatry setting as (moral) reasons for responding in certain ways and for instilling certain virtues in the character of the practitioner. Although we do not defend it here, we follow many in contemporary meta-ethics in adhering to a version of moral realism. As such, we eschew ethical subjectivism and relativism and locate moral truths outside the subject.[2]

Similarly, although this is a book about character and the self, we presuppose rather than defend our conception of the person as an enduring, defining, and integrated metaphysical entity.[3] While this more abstract notion plays little part in our argument, we do place extensive reliance on what is sometimes distinguished as "characterization" identity (Schechtman 1996). A person's characterization identity is constituted by the content of her socially constructed self-concept. It includes, for example, her gender identity and the attributes by which she is known to others and defines herself. We also introduce Korsgaard's notion of "practical identity" when we are explaining the normative force of identity-conferring social roles such as that of being a doctor.

Cases are introduced to elucidate our discussions in the following chapters. This material was derived from experience in clinical settings. Suitably disguised, these cases portray real, particular contingencies. Still, they suffer some of the drawbacks that have recently been noted in all conventional ethics case narratives (Chambers 1999). They are post hoc depictions of static "moments," distorted and oversimplified by the heuristic purposes they serve. In an attempt to remedy some of these narrative limitations, a final chapter has been added (Chapter 7) that allows the reader to better experience the dynamic ebb and flow of the extended sequence of a therapeutic exchange. A stream of consciousness narrative is employed that, in keeping with the virtue ethics emphasis on inner states as well as their outer expression, exposes some of the practitioner's felt responses and silent monologue.

The prescriptive conclusions of this book are few and simple. Psychiatry should be recognized to have its own ethics, whose strictures function as a

[2] For an overview of these positions see Miller (2003).
[3] For a fuller account of these questions of personal or self-identity, see Radden (1996, 2004).

complement to the other moral demands on practitioners derived from bio-medical ethics. A character-focused virtue ethics framework will best fulfill this demand. It should be adopted. And along with other practice skills, trainee practitioners ought to be helped to acquire the added virtue and extra virtues called for by the practice setting.

*

We have situated our explorations within several different research lit-eratures, and tried to build on the work of others—within moral philosophy and psychology, bioethics, social psychology, moral education, and psychi-atry itself. Much in the following pages represents original analysis as well, however, and the chapter summaries that follow provide some indication of where our approach, or the substance of our findings, break new ground.

In Chapter 1 we acknowledge past research, locating psychiatric ethics within professional and biomedical ethics more generally understood. Then "role morality" is introduced, vis., the notion that some ethical imperatives derive from particular social roles. By analyzing a case example we show some of the ways psychiatry seems to differ from most other medical prac-tices. The case also indicates the particular focus of our claims: psychiatry practiced with those suffering severe mental disorders. Three specific areas revealing such differences are introduced: questions of patient autonomy, the "boundaries" of the therapeutic relationship and concerns over psychi-atric diagnostic categories. We identify the approach adopted, including our attitude toward the much-vaunted contemporary model of the psychiatric patient as a consumer of services. This chapter builds on work in biomedical ethics, and adopts the methodology employed in the American Psychiatric Association's *Annotations with Particular Application to Psychiatry* (2001), in which the ethical implications of particular features distinctive to the practice of psychiatry are identified.

An explanation and defense of our emphasis on the way psychiatry is different are put forward in Chapter 2. We argue that although few aspects of the practice are unique to it, taken together a set of elements constitutes psy-chiatry as a unique healing practice. Features such as patient vulnerability, attitudes toward psychiatric symptoms, stigma, and controversy over mental disorder in our culture, and the nature of the therapeutic project in psy-chiatry are explored, together with more recent factors influencing practice: managed care delivery systems and the advent of the consumer movements. Previous research has been centered on one or another feature distinguishing the psychiatry setting (issues of classification and diagnosis, or involuntary treatment, for example). By focusing on assorted aspects of the setting that jointly distinguish it, and showing the way they provide moral reasons for practitioners, our discussion breaks new ground. The often resisted or over-looked view that psychiatry requires its own ethics is thus provided with a systematic and developed rationale.

Chapter 3 introduces the notion of psychiatric ethics understood as virtue ethics. We show why a virtue ethics framework suits the role morality associated with professionalism and introduce the category of a role-constituted virtue. The latter is called for by the practice setting because of its conduciveness to healing. We explain how applications of virtue ethics to practice can avoid vagueness and a reduction to platitudes, and offer reasons why a virtue ethics framework particularly fits psychiatric practice. This chapter builds on contemporary philosophical writing on virtue theory, especially that of Oakley and Cocking (2001). The original contribution of the chapter lies in its explication of the character demands of the psychiatry setting. Not only the special importance of what we have called unruly virtues, which elude rule-based approaches, and those virtues such as moral leadership that are supererogatory, but other aspects of the moral psychology of virtue-focused systems are recognized and provided original analyses here. These findings will have broader application, we believe, laying the groundwork for any thoroughly worked out neo-Aristotelian, biomedical ethics.

Gender has been introduced in Chapter 2, with reference to today's emphasis on characterization identity; it is also the focus in Chapter 4, where the centrality of gender to psychiatry and to the psychiatric project is demonstrated. (These include the cultural associations linking male heterosexuality with mental health, the bias found in diagnostic categories, the differential treatment provided to women, and the implications of practicing psychiatry within traditionally male-oriented cultures.) Moving beyond questions about misogyny, homophobia, and homosexuality to explore the ethics of practice with transgendered identities, we outline the elements of a gender-sensitive psychiatry. As one implication of recent identity politics, issues of gender identity represent an inescapable ethical challenge for today's practitioner and reflect ideas that have received little systematic attention. More generally, our stress on the controversial and central place of gender within psychiatric lore and practice is one that is developed and supported here more thoroughly than in almost all other research, and our exploration into the implication of these features of psychiatry for practice that is gender sensitive, similarly, is entirely new to the present work.

A sampling of the virtues called for by the psychiatric setting is enumerated in Chapter 5. Several different kinds of character traits are included here: some, such as trustworthiness and moral integrity, are moral virtues as essential in everyday as professional life. Some others, while elsewhere merely prudential or intellectual virtues, become role-constituted virtues for the practitioner in psychiatry. (Propriety and realism are examples.) Finally, some traits are closely role-constituted virtues, such as unselfing and propriety. They seem to be without universally recognized moral value outside of the professional setting.

This is not intended to be a complete portrait of the character of the virtuous psychiatrist. Rather, it is a template for identifying that character by appeal to particular aspects of the psychiatry setting. The virtues named above, as well as a handful of others (gender sensitivity, the moral leadership demanded by managed care psychiatry, empathy, patience, and fortitude, self-knowledge and self-unity, respectfulness, and the metavirtues of authenticity and *phronesis*) are each analyzed individually in an effort to demonstrate their link to demands determined by that setting.

Philosophical research in moral psychology from the last two decades provides the foundation for the detailed analysis of each of the virtues we undertake here. But here, too, we have extended the discussion in a number of ways. The hitherto unacknowledged practitioner's trait of unselfing (defined as the personally effaced yet acutely attentive and affectively attuned attitude toward the patient, the relationship, and its boundaries, adopted by the ethical and effective practitioner), introduces an entirely new concept. The discussion of propriety as a trait required of the practitioner because of the public safety powers bestowed upon him or her, applies the concept of appearance standards to a completely different setting. More generally, the emphasis on the communicative skills required to *convey*—and not merely possess—the virtues demanded by the psychiatry setting represents an emphasis not found in other writing.

In Chapter 6 we expose certain difficulties associated with adopting a virtue-focused framework for a professional ethics. Tensions inherent in wedding the traditional concept of character to that of social roles are illustrated through the moral dangers associated with inner compartmentalization, inconstant virtues, and incompatible roles (such as healer and upholder of criminal justice). We also note some difficulties springing from the way virtues are habituated, evaluating the moral status of virtues that are merely feigned. This enumeration and discussion of the tensions involved in combining virtue ethics and role morality have implications for any professional ethics where such a combination seems so apposite. Apart from advancing understanding within moral psychology, then, the explorations in this chapter represent a contribution to professional ethics more generally understood.

Chapter 7 brings together the themes of the previous chapters. It comprises a series of detailed cases that illustrate some of the points developed previously and demonstrate our emphasis on the moral psychology and character of the practitioner. Although at root they remain illustrative fictions or "just so" stories, and are amalgams from the clinical experience of Sadler and his colleagues, these narratives aim to capture the inner world of the practitioner as well as the dynamic ebb and flow of the interchange between patient(s) and practitioner during particular "moments" in the therapeutic session.

Finally, in a brief concluding chapter, we return to the question of whether, and how, virtue can be taught, first introduced in Chapter 5. We point to a growing body of evidence indicating it is possible to deepen and augment the affective and moral responses making up character traits such as empathy using a range of pedagogical techniques that harness imaginative capabilities. Alongside the practice skills learned, we propose that the virtues of the good practitioner in psychiatry should be taught and focus should be directed to the trainees' character.

*

The authorship and division of labor here reflects the project's dual foci of moral psychology and philosophy, on the one hand, and the particulars of practice, on the other. One author (Radden) is an academic philosopher with a long interest in the moral and philosophical implications of mental health issues. The other author (Sadler) is a philosophically skilled clinician with many years of practice and an academic focus in medical ethics. Philosophical insights must be tethered to clinical realities, and the following collaborative effort represents a sustained, cross-disciplinary exploration, in which philosophical grounding and practice bring, we hope, genuine synergy.

1 Psychiatric Ethics as Professional and Biomedical Ethics

There is no fun in psychiatry. If you try to get fun out of it, you pay a considerable price. If you do not feel equal to the headaches that psychiatry induces, you are in the wrong business.

HARRY STACK SULLIVAN, THE PSYCHIATRIC INTERVIEW (1954: 10)

Introduction

Psychiatry is an exacting practice. It is no fun, as Sullivan suggests, and headache-inducing. We believe the demands on the practitioner in psychiatry are moral or ethical as well as technical. One of the main themes of this book is that the moral demands on psychiatrists go beyond those imposed by the medical and professional roles they inhabit. But this chapter starts with the demands that are shared with other doctors, and even with other professionals.

As one among many forms of biomedical practice, psychiatry is governed by the same ethical principles as any medical subspeciality, be it surgery, internal medicine, obstetrics, or urology. Explored, clarified, and refined within the last several decades of the twentieth century, these principles include articulated values and ideals, such as respect for autonomy, which can be used to guide ethical practice. The classic statement of these principles is found in Tom Beauchamp and James Childress's *Principles of Biomedical Ethics* (fifth edition 2001). Here, autonomy, nonmaleficence (*primum non nocere*), beneficence, and justice are represented as core, shared values. Although they are each action-guiding, the principles of autonomy, nonmaleficence, beneficence, and justice are not ranked in any systematic way, and they often conflict in practice settings.

Because the principles enumerated by Beauchamp and Childress are not formally ranked, ethical decision making is represented as a discursive activity: proceeding case by case, it calls for deliberation, consultation, and judgment. They may conflict in application to particular situations, but the four principles of autonomy, nonmaleficence, beneficence, and justice form the frame within which bioethical decision making can be conducted. They provide, in Beauchamp's words, a "starting point" for moral judgment and policy evaluation (Beauchamp 1999: 33).

This principle-based approach has long dominated biomedical ethics.[1] It is intended for, and aptly applies to, all medical specialities, including psychiatry.

Psychiatry is situated within the family of medically related practices governed by the principles of biomedical ethics outlined above. These principles are encoded in formal statements such as that of the American Medical Association (AMA 2000). Biomedicine is, in turn, nested within and answerable to the moral and ethical ideals guiding all the professions (Agich 1980; Flexner 1915; Metzger 1975; Ozar 1995; Pellegrino 1979; Pellegrino and Thomasma 1993; Sadler 2005).

Many ethical demands have been seen as shared across professional practices. Dentists, accountants, teachers, and lawyers—as much as doctors—recognize professional codes of conduct ensuring that they behave honorably, and respect the fundamental, contractual relationship between provider and recipient of professional services. Professional status in this broad sense has been identified in terms of traits such as trustworthiness, fidelity, honesty, and integrity. To have a profession distinct from having mere technique, it has been said, implies: "the possession of certain character-defining traits or qualities" (Kronman 1987: 841). (Although trustworthiness, fidelity, honesty, and integrity are the traits or qualities most commonly cited as called for by every professional setting, another obvious quality is the Aristotelian virtue of *phronesis*, generally translated as "practical wisdom." *Phronesis* seems to be as necessary for the ethical practice of law, or even

---

[1] It has been challenged, of course. Supporters of utilitarianism, of a more traditional deontological and Kantian approach, of various forms of virtue ethics, feminist and narrative approaches, and/or an ethics of care, have each found reasons to criticize the theory and application of Beauchamp and Childress's approach (Beauchamp 1995; Bloch and Green 2006; Clouser and Gert 1994; Gert et al. 1997; Lustig 1992; Veatch 2003).

business, as medicine: any professional practice will require the combined grasp of particulars, astuteness, perception, and understanding making up *phronesis*, which direct us toward right action.)

The doctor's particular professional role is as healer, however, and the principles governing professional conduct would not alone be sufficient to address the ethical demands of that role. The principles of professional ethics must be amplified and amended to acknowledge the distinctive practice of medicine. From its beginnings in the West, such a practice has been recognized to impose its own special ethical constraints. For example, the Hippocratic *primum non nocere* has particular bearing for the doctor because, unlike other professionals, the doctor wields authority over a recipient of professional services (the patient) who is made needy and vulnerable by illness, disability, and perhaps danger to life.

The psychiatrist has at least two sets of ethical obligations, then. As a professional, she has duties and responsibilities stemming from her role as a provider of professional services. As a doctor she honors the more particular ethical guidelines applicable to the practice of all medicine.

This much has long been acknowledged. Our argument in this book is that the psychiatrist has a third set of ethical obligations, in addition to those imposed by her professional status and by her status as a doctor. This third set of obligations is imposed by the specialty of psychiatry itself, and is called for by aspects of the psychiatric practice setting. Commonalities across medical practice, and even the shared ideals framing every professional endeavor, unite psychiatrists with other practitioners and professionals; about this there can be no doubt. But it is our contention that just as the principles of professional ethics are alone insufficient to govern the distinctive practice of medicine, the principles or ethical rules governing all medical subspecialties do not completely account for ethical dilemmas and challenges arising within psychiatric care. These dilemmas and challenges require qualifications on and additions to standard biomedical ethics. They impose added constraints, concerns, and responsibilities on—and, we argue, call for particular virtues in the characters of—psychiatric practitioners.

While they are also found in other areas of medical practice, some of these constraints, concerns, and responsibilities are nonetheless more common in the practice of psychiatry. Others are apparently magnified and intensified by that practice. Only one feature of the psychiatric setting may be entirely unique to it: among medical practitioners, psychiatrists alone always have laws empowering them, and often, only them, to seclude and treat nonconsenting patients. This factor in itself, we emphasize, imposes a distinctive mark on the character of the psychiatrist and demands special ethical responses fitted to the unique social role involved. Yet, while this may be the sole feature of psychiatry that is entirely distinct to it, a collection of other features, in combination, serve to distinguish psychiatry as a unique social and medical practice.

Some simple examples can introduce those features of psychiatric practice that impose ethical demands exceeding those imposed within other medical settings—features explored more fully in later chapters. Consider, then (i) A group as apparently vulnerable to exploitation as psychiatric patients might require exceptional forbearance and self-discipline on the part of the psychiatrist. (ii) Disorders so dependent on the communication of symptoms and, at the same time, apt to interfere with communicative capabilities will require great patience, compassion, and understanding from the practitioner. (iii) Symptoms as regularly painless and even pleasurable as those of some mental disorders, such as mania, encourage complex and ambivalent attitudes in those experiencing them, and these attitudes will likely demand additional vigilance, and extra perseverance, on the part of practitioners. (iv) Because mental disorder is still controversial and subject to misunderstanding and stigma, the intimate, personal and private details regularly explored in treatment will almost certainly call for extra trustworthiness and care over confidentiality. (v) Disorders so frequently affecting their sufferers' autonomy, mood, and reasoning capabilities—the traits associated with personhood—will likely call for extra moral seriousness and effort. (vi) As arbiter over our society's central values of autonomy and rationality, the psychiatrist is "moralist" (Rieff 1959) as well as healer, and this role seems to call for judgment beyond the ordinary in practitioners and perhaps even gravitas, or wisdom. (vii) The psychiatrist is vested by society with the unique power of restraining and treating adults against their wishes not only for the sake of others' safety but also for their own—a power calling for a special degree of moral integrity in those who exercise it.

Because our argument for a distinctive ethic for psychiatry is developed within a virtue ethics framework, we have chosen to express the handful of brief examples provided in list (i)–(vii) in terms of particular traits located in the practitioner's character. But the demands shown in these examples might equally have been depicted in terms of extra duties and responsibilities incumbent in the practitioner's role.

The reasoning in what follows mirrors the schematic approach employed in these seven examples: aspects of the psychiatry setting are shown to call for particular ethical responses in practitioners that go considerably beyond the responsibilities, duties, and character virtues imposed by their status as professionals, and even as doctors. A few of the examples listed in (i)–(vii), such as the demand for greater confidentiality in the psychiatry setting are unarguable, and widely accepted; others may be more controversial—although, through the course of this book, we hope to show their force.

On account of the higher standard prescribed in this reasoning, however, we want to begin with some clarification of the implications of this "psychiatric exceptionalism."

Opportunities for Unethical Behavior

> Insofar as all those who come to him must be by definition relatively insecure, the psychiatrist is peculiarly estopped from seeking personal satisfactions or prestige at their expense. (Harry Stack Sullivan 1954: 12)

Several of the examples listed in (i)–(vii) illustrate ways in which the psychiatric setting permits or even invites unethical conduct on the part of the practitioner. The opportunity to exploit the patient and to succumb to the temptations provided by the patient's vulnerabilities and neediness point to extra moral care and concern required in this setting. It may be true that equality arising from a balanced distribution of power is the very safest remedy against the tendency to harmful exploitation inherent in any relationship between the weak and the powerful (Goodin 1988; Wertheimer 1996).[2] But another remedy is a suitably stringent ethical code—or a virtuous character. (In fact, we argue in Chapter 3, both these are necessary: the virtuous

---

[2] Political philosopher Robert Goodin has named four conditions, all of which must be present if dependencies are to be exploitable; arguably, the psychiatry setting is characterized in varying degrees and at different times by all four. First, the relationship must be asymmetrical; second, "the subordinate party must *need* the resource that the superordinate supplies"; third "the subordinate party must depend upon some *particular* subordinate for the supply of needed resources"; fourth, "the superordinate enjoys discretionary control over the resources that the subordinate needs from him" (Goodin 1988: 37).

character supplements and augments ethical rules with its emphasis on personal accountability and on the appropriate moral psychology—not just doing the right thing, but doing it for the right reason, for example.)

The vulnerabilities associated with patients in no way imply that practitioners in psychiatry are more exploitative than other professionals (any more than child protection laws cast aspersions on the character of parents as a group). In fact, rather the contrary may be true: given the magnitude of the opportunities for unethical behavior practitioners in psychiatry seem to us to be, for the most part, admirably honorable, trustworthy, and restrained. But the psychiatry setting is one whose arrangements—including a completely private meeting wherein intimate and personal details about one but not the other of the two parties are the center of a discussion designedly free of restraint—accords unchecked power to the practitioner. Because of this, it allows and even invites exploitative responses, if not ingrained vices. As Alan Wertheimer has observed, "the modality of psychotherapeutic treatment puts the psychotherapist at considerable 'risk' of becoming an exploiter" (Wertheimer 1996: 159).

Psychiatrists must sometimes repel active and open seductiveness from patients in settings of the utmost privacy, for example. Moreover, they must do so without conveying personal rejection, losing the patient's trust, or otherwise damaging, compromising, or jeopardizing the therapeutic relationship. Against such temptations any person would likely require special protection: not just extra external rules and restrictions but also more deeply internalized rules, greater self-control, and other character virtues.

Practitioners do not always succeed in this and like endeavors, perhaps not surprisingly. But that they sometimes fall short does not detract from the point made here: the ethical challenge such endeavors present, and the ethical demands they impose.

To say this is not to diminish the egregious nature of these sexual predations and the importance of their detection and censure. Much attention has been paid to the dangers of, and resulting damage from, sexual misconduct perpetrated on patients by practitioners. Moreover, codified rules and penalties have rightly been devised to prevent and punish such conduct (Appelbaum and Jorgenson 1991; Edelwich and Brodsky 1991; Freeman and Roy 1976; Gabbard 1989; Gantrell 1994). There are dangers besides the temptation to engage in sexual misconduct, however. Perhaps less obvious, these temptations include the satisfactions derived from invidious comparison— feeling superior or more fortunate in contrast to those less well positioned than ourselves; from "playing God" out of a perceived greater appreciation of another person's (here, the patient's) best interests; from taking a prurient interest in, or vicarious enjoyment over, another person's intimate and personal story; and finally, and more generally, from the human tendency to indulge bias, whimsy, arbitrariness, and prejudice, and the inclination to preserve self-esteem and psychological unity at the expense of the other person.

Many of these temptations derive from traits that are part of human nature and attributable to all of us—some even reflect traditional vices, such as pride. Additional, and different, temptations arise from the practitioner's status. James Drane argues that the power and respect all physicians enjoy places them at special risk of self-ignorance and self-deception. Because of their position of authority in the modern, medical delivery system, he notes, doctors "can easily come to think that they are always right and, consequently, ignore their deep-seated fallibility" (Drane 1995: 61). Another kind of temptation is driven by the model of psychiatrist as mere technical expert. We consider misplaced the modesty of embracing such a limited professional identity. Comforting, and tempting as it may be, as we show in Chapters 5 and 6, this way of construing the psychiatrist's role is insufficient, and incompatible with the respect for the therapeutic project called for by the psychiatry setting.

Occasions to act on temptations and desires like the ones identified here are as much part of psychiatric practice as are occasions inviting the more commonly acknowledged vices. And because all the above temptations are a customary part of psychiatric practice, the moral demands on the practitioner will be comparably great.

Role Morality

The practitioner in psychiatry has a set of nested ethical obligations deriving from her status and role as a professional, as a doctor, and finally as a psychiatrist. The relationship between these differing obligations can best be illustrated by introducing the concept of role morality. Role morality refers to a set of obligations or constraints attaching to, and generated by, a particular social role. Our practitioner's role as a professional entails some of these—she must be honest, for example. Her role as a doctor imposes further obligations—like all medical practitioners, she must treat her patient mindful of what is most conducive to health and healing. And finally, her role as psychiatrist obliges her to care for the patient's psychological well-being.

Role morality is understood in a weaker and less controversial form, and a stronger and more controversial form. Weak role morality is implicit in any claim made for a distinctive professional ethics: it will impose on anyone undertaking particular professional roles additional rules of conduct more specifically applied than, yet apparently compatible with, the obligations imposed by broad-based morality. Because this sort of role morality refers to more, not less, stringent obligations than those of broad-based morality, its dictates are uncontroversial. These two sets of obligations are not in conflict: the demands of weak role morality never override, they only add to, the dictates of broad-based morality. The role of the doctor will serve to illustrate here. Following Hippocratic teaching even consenting sexual relations between unmarried, adult doctors and their unmarried, adult patients are forbidden. Yet broad-based morality (in much of Western liberal democratic culture, at least) permits such relationships between consenting, unmarried adults. The more stringent demands imposed on the doctor, because they are compatible with the looser ones of broad-based morality, represent an instance of weak role morality.

Strong role morality is more controversial. It asserts that what is morally permissible or even morally required by, for instance, a professional role, is not even permitted on the broad-based morality applicable to the rest of the society. Even if some action conflicts with the moral rules expressing broad-based morality, role morality for the doctor is dictated by the goal of maintaining or restoring the patient's health. Confronted by a wounded, dangerous, fleeing convict, it might be said, the doctor's duty differs from other citizens': he is bound to treat the wounds before, or even instead of, assisting in the man's capture, as broad-based morality would dictate. (As this example illustrates, role morality rests on the assumption that broad-based morality contains tenets adhered to by all, such as the citizen's duty to assist in law enforcement. This assumption may be challenged, of course, although it is an innocuous one in the present discussion. For a recent discussion of its warrant, see Beauchamp [1999] and Veatch [2003].)[3]

---

[3] Another example of strong role morality might be that of the subterfuges employed by trial lawyers. Although apparently called for by the zealous advocacy that is part of the lawyer's professional role, such conduct arguably contravenes the directives of broad-based morality, with its high standard of communicative transparency and plain dealing.

The form of role morality employed in the discussions that follow is for the most part the less controversial, weak role morality, which simply adds to, rather than contravening the dictates of broad-based morality. One virtue that arguably introduces stronger role morality is unselfing, discussed in Chapter 5. But although they *may* contravene some social norms, we show, even the traits making up unselfing fail to violate broad-based morality.

Finding an Appropriate Model

Endemic to much practice, research, managed mental health care, and today's consumer advocacy movements is a model of the psychiatric patient. In this model the patient is a client or consumer, an autonomous agent capable of giving or withholding informed consent for treatment, and able to contract for psychiatric services (Radden 2008; Rhodes 2005). Close observers of the profession recognized the emergence of this model before the last decade of the twentieth century (Benatar 1987; Emanuel and Emanuel 1992, Frank and Frank 1991; Veatch 1991). Writing in 1991, Jerome and Julia Frank noted the increasingly popular use of terms borrowed from business and law, which they saw as a trend influenced by the growing role of third party payers who analogize psychotherapy to "a contract for the provision of services," where "psychotherapists are called providers, patients are labeled consumers of a product called mental health care, and their interactions are guided by a therapeutic contract specifying the obligations and rewards of both parties" (Frank and Frank 1991: 180).

These commentators could hardly have guessed the power and influence of the trend they identified. Today, the consumer model is so favored that it has eclipsed other, earlier models. Biomedical ethics, managed care medicine, much biological psychiatry, and the mental health consumers' movements, are in spectacular accord in their embrace of this depiction of the psychiatric patient as consumer.

The consumer model is an attractive one, for psychiatric patients and practitioners alike. Practitioners' knowledge and skill on this model are a commodity like any other; a commodity that the consumer wants, and for which he or she is able to negotiate a fair exchange. This relationship transforms the practitioner from a paternalistic healer to a professional expert analogous to other professionals providing expertise and special skills to their clients, and meeting those clients on equal terms.

As this suggests, the new relationship offers much. It involves an exchange that is mutually advantageous between practitioner and client or consumer. It presupposes reciprocal respect and a shared understanding between the two parties. It is a relationship that depends on mutual trust. And it is one that upholds the fundamentally egalitarian notion that the consumer is endowed with roughly equal social power, and is able to use it to further her own interests. Autonomy and the trait of self-reliance; mutuality and mutual respect; equality and egalitarianism; trust and trustworthiness— these are all widely valued principles and traits that seem integral to the consumer model.

Despite the powerful convergence of opinion in favor of the consumer model, and the fact that the presumption of autonomy is a mainstay of our society's liberal democratic *ethos*, the applicability of the model within the psychiatry setting cannot be adopted on faith. Because psychiatric patients are often deprived—if only temporarily and partially—of the very capabilities required for an exercise of autonomy, the appropriateness of the consumer model for psychiatric practice, and particularly its successful eclipse of other models, deserve much closer scrutiny. For, arguably, it occludes and betrays some of what is most central to ethical psychiatric practice.

Consider that such a model presupposes that the consumer always acts freely and knowingly, understanding her options and their implications, and is able to examine these in light of her long-term goals and interests. It presupposes that a rough social equality pertains between the purveyor of services and the consumer of those services in the power each has vis à vis what the other wants. It presupposes a certain mutuality of purpose and understanding between the purveyor of services and the consumer of those services, which includes agreement over whether there is a problem, what the problem is, what remedies are appropriate for the problem, and the roles of each participant. It presupposes that once a level of basic trust is established, the relationship between purveyor and consumer of services is well nigh incidental to the effectiveness of the transaction—an effectiveness measured solely, or almost solely, by the skill of the expert. Yet when it comes to the psychiatric patient, none of these features is unfailingly present. (These tensions over the consumer model, it should be added, were also recognized early. Frank and Frank commented that the basic flaw of the consumer model was the assumption that "like partners in a business deal, both parties to the therapeutic contract are free, autonomous agents" [Frank and Frank 1991: 180].)

Writing in the 1980s, Paul McHugh and Philip Slavney were able to dismiss the call to refer to patients as clients as arising from "wishful thinking and … a sentimental and superficial understanding of psychiatric disorders and a desire to avoid the responsibilities of a physician to those in his care" (McHugh and Slavney 1987: 96). Today, we recognize this inquiry into the applicability of the consumer model to be an infinitely more serious and delicate one than that passage deriding the name change suggests. The modern day promotion and presumption of autonomy have been tools to undo the ill effects of past stigmatizing and prejudicial attitudes, attitudes that, too often, have entirely denied to psychiatric patients all rational capabilities and, on that basis, any autonomy. Moreover, as was noted above, the voices of patients themselves are often raised loudest in insisting on their recognition as autonomous "consumers" of mental health services—rather than the suffering, hapless victims of their disease. By approaching the patient's breakdown in terms of illness, disability and dysfunction, as one such service user has put it, "the system has consistently underestimated my capacity to change and has ignored the potential it may contain to assist that change. My desire to win my own control of the breakdown process and thereby to gain independence and integrity has not only been ignored—it has been thwarted" (Campbell 1996: 56–57).

It must be possible to acknowledge and avoid the wrongs associated with the cruel and discriminatory attitudes of the past without resorting to a misapplication of the consumer model, however.[4] And unwarrantedly attributing capabilities to the psychiatric patient when such capabilities are compromised involves an injustice paralleling that involved in denying autonomy when it is present.

An inquiry into which is more appropriate within the psychiatry setting, "sick patient" or "autonomous consumer," is complicated in two ways. One complication is raised by the range of cases seen by psychiatrists, from extremely disordered and needy people who are clearly sick patients, to those more aptly described—and increasingly insistent upon describing themselves—as autonomous clients or consumers. In addition, however, the question is also complicated by the nature, and course, of the illness

---

[4] It may not be entirely possible without revision of some of the individualistic presuppositions underlying traditional conception of autonomy. As contemporary critics have shown, the "autonomous self" is in many ways a misleading fiction (Christman 2004; Christman and Anderson 2006; Friedman 2003). See also Card (1991), Meyers (1997), and Brennan (1999: 868–872).

experience itself, which is replete, in most psychiatric disorders, with stages and phases varying widely on this dimension. The main focus of the present book is settings where patients are treated for severe mental disorders. But even sick patients at one point in their treatment process will likely become autonomous consumers at another. Of this wide and dynamic range characterizing severe psychiatric disorders, Deborah Spitz observes: "They are chronic, characterized by relapses and periods of respite. The patient goes through episodes of incapacity and episodes of clarity, times of disorganization, psychosis, hopelessness and dependency and other periods of cogency, reflection, and collaborative planning. The relationship between psychiatrist and patient shifts to mirror the changes in the patient's illness; neither the disease nor the doctor-patient relationship is static" (Spitz 1996: 238).

In Chapter 2, we look more closely at the recipient of psychiatric services together with the project of healing in psychiatry and try to determine whether, and when, "sick patient" or "autonomous consumer" better accords with what we see. But we do so recognizing that not one or the other but both models, sick patient and autonomous consumer, will have a place in the psychiatric setting.

Annotations Especially Applicable to Psychiatry

Biomedical ethics is itself young, for the most part it is the product of the last decades of the twentieth century.[5] And that same period has seen much focused attention on the evaluative norms undergirding the practice, theory, and knowledge base of psychiatry. Psychiatric ethics, understood as an attempt to codify and proscribe for psychiatric practice, is even younger (Musto 1999). Moreover, much writing about ethical psychiatric practice draws attention to the commonalities uniting the psychiatrist with other biomedical specialists and, as such, with other professionals. Less attention has been paid to the dissimilarities.

That along with their responsibilities and duties derived from professional ethics and from biomedical ethics, psychiatrists will need additional guidance and their own particular *ethos* has, from time to time, been acknowledged. Much important research in the last two decades has also paved the way for thinking about the ethical quandaries and moral dilemmas distinctive to, or at least greatly magnified by, the psychiatric setting.

---

[5] Some notable exceptions include the medical ethics associated with theological writing, and the work of Percival (Percival 1803).

This writing, by Bloch and Chodoff (1981), Bloch et al. (1999), Dunn (1998), Dickenson and Fulford (2000), Dyer (1988, 1999), Edwards (1982, 1997), Fulford (1989), Fulford et al. (2003), Martin (2001), Reiser et al. (1987), Radden (1996, 2002a, 2002b, 2004), and Sadler (2005), among others, explored and clarified a range of fundamental ethical issues arising in psychiatry. In particular, a substantial and valuable literature is focused on (1) the patient's decisional capacity and involuntary treatment; (2) the rules governing the conduct of the therapeutic relationship; and (3) the controversial aspects of psychiatric classification and diagnosis—all three topics introduced later in the present chapter.

As well as the above contributions, there is an important source that acknowledges the distinctiveness of psychiatric practice and offers ethical guidelines particular to psychiatry. This comes to us as amendments to the American Medical Association's Code of Medical Ethics provided by the American Psychiatric Association (APA 2001). First published in 1973, these *Annotations Especially Applicable to Psychiatry* have been expanded and altered over the years to reflect changes and developments in APA thinking about ethical issues as they arose in the actual, difficult cases within psychiatric practice brought to the attention of the Association's Ethics Committees.

In spite of these changes and accretions, the principle behind the *Annotations* has remained unchanged; it rests on an explicit acknowledgment that while psychiatrists and other physicians share goals, "there are special ethical problems in psychiatric practice." These problems "differ in *coloring and degree* from the ethical problems in other branches of medical practice, even though the basic principles are the same" (APA 2001: 02, our emphasis). The *Annotations* go on to indicate particular features of psychiatric practice giving rise to ethical responsibilities more stringent than those imposed by the principles of the American Medical Association in its code. Although its account of these features is brief and unsystematic, the *Annotations*' portrayal of the special features of psychiatric practice provides a useful exemplar for our approach in this and the following chapters. To ascertain what is distinctive to psychiatric ethics, the *Annotations* method proceeds by considering what is distinctive to the practice of psychiatry. Only when that uniqueness has been identified and explored, it is assumed, will we possess the foundation necessary for recognizing the ethical psychiatrist and ethical practice within psychiatry.

Several features of psychiatric practice have been noted and emphasized in the *Annotations*. The same features also appear in the body of research and writing with implications for psychiatric ethics noted earlier, although the latter writing is not always as explicit as the *Annotations* in acknowledging the relationship between features of practice and an ethics for psychiatry.

In Chapter 2 we engage in a more thoroughgoing defense of the claim that the practice of psychiatry differs sufficiently from other medical practices to require an ethics over and above that imposed on its practitioners by dint of their status as professionals and as medical doctors. In the remainder of this chapter we explore the three aspects of the practice setting—each emblematic of the uniqueness of psychiatry—that are identified as points (1)–(3) above. These serve to highlight what the *Annotations* describe as the distinctive "coloring and degree" of its ethical problems. The first of these concerns patient autonomy and a case example illustrates the way psychiatric practice seems to sharpen and magnify the customary tensions around respecting the autonomy of patients. The second is the therapeutic relationship or alliance between patient and practitioner, which has given rise to the special language and rules governing the preservation of "boundaries" in the therapeutic setting. The third is the taxonomy underpinning diagnosis, the controversy surrounding which in psychiatry is unprecedented. In contrast to many of the features introduced in Chapter 2, each of these three topics (patient autonomy; the therapeutic relationship; psychiatric diagnostic categories and diagnosis) has received considerable, although isolated, attention from those writing about biomedical ethics in application to psychiatry.

Patient Autonomy: Case Example

Some of the dilemmas and problems around patient autonomy that are so distinctively psychiatric can be most readily revealed through a case example.

> An adult patient with paranoid schizophrenia has discontinued her antipsychotic medication and has threatened her aging parents at knifepoint because "they are the toxin people who want me to be a good girl." Her parents obtained a mental illness warrant (court order) for a brief psychiatric evaluation, and you, her long-standing doctor, are familiar with the following clinical pattern. She will agree to resume taking her medication to stay out of the hospital, but not follow through with this commitment until involuntarily hospitalized and medicated back to her baseline nondelusional

state. The patient's parents are urging you to again seclude the patient without her consent. Moreover, the managed care reviewer who would permit reimbursement for care refuses to "certify" (endorse) hospital care because "the patient is willing to take medication as an outpatient."

This case raises many questions. Most broadly, is this patient rightly seen as an autonomous person, a rational agent capable of determining her own interests, an informed consumer of medical services, and one able to enter into an agreement about taking medication as an outpatient? How, more generally, should the parents' physical safety be balanced against the patient's individual rights? Indeed, given the hardships of living with a schizophrenia sufferer, how should the parents' interests and stake in this decision be ranked against the patient's own? Ought the practitioner's prediction of outcome be honored over the assessment proffered by the managed care reviewer? How do we regard the professional role conflicts imposed on the psychiatrist, who is caught between the goals of ensuring safety for the parents and the patient, maintaining the critical "alliance" with the patient necessary for any long-term therapeutic success, and using whatever means to reduce her dangerous, delusional thinking?

Some of these dilemmas and difficulties, or closely related ones, may have complements in other specialties of medicine; others have none, or at least very, very few analogies in other medical fields. And, as this example illustrates, these are quandaries amplified, rather than reduced, by managed care medicine.

The principles governing all biomedical ethics are undeniably useful for the practitioner dealing with cases such as this one. Clearly, the value of autonomy, a principle accepted not only throughout medical but throughout professional ethics, will have to be part of any deliberation over ethical conduct in such a case, as will that of beneficence. And, as is so often true throughout biomedical ethics, patient autonomy and beneficence appear to be in tension here, presenting a common quandary or dilemma for the practitioner. Even the commitment to the principle of justice might be seen to be implicated in this complex decision. The patient's apparent rights—to refuse her treatment, and to be trusted and respected in her predicted bargain— might be seen to introduce one kind of obligation for the person treating her. But the principle of beneficence, reflected in the practitioner's recognition that her patient's decisional capabilities can be enhanced with medication, is also pertinent—added to which the impulse to help her and ensure the family's safety has its own legitimacy. On balance, preventing the danger to others posed by the untreated patient may present itself as a duty stemming from the principle of justice. The ethical decision here can be portrayed as one of balancing, competing, and incompatible goods or duties, and it will be a difficult and weighty, though painfully familiar, one.

Leaving the analysis at this point, however, would be failing to acknowledge the extent that this case is typical, even emblematic, of psychiatric ethical dilemmas. What distinguishes our practitioner's dilemma from conflicts around the value of autonomy within the rest of biomedical ethics is that the tensions seem more starkly etched here. The issue is not merely whether to honor the patient's autonomy over the principles of beneficence, nonmaleficence, or justice, but whether the category of autonomy is applicable at all. Even when, with every appearance of self-interested rationality, the patient tries to bargain with her doctor, promising to take her medicine if in return she need not return to the hospital, the nature of her illness forces us to ask whether the attempted agreement is a genuine expression of rational processes and personal decision.[6]

Therapeutic "Boundaries"

The *Annotations* indicate several features of the therapeutic relationship in psychiatry giving rise to ethical responsibilities more stringent than those imposed by the American Medical Association Code of Ethics. Three of these are of particular importance to our discussion. (1) The therapeutic relationship is vital to effective treatment. (2) The relationship and the treatment it effects involve matters so private, personal, and emotional that the patient is especially vulnerable to both exploitation and breaches of confidentiality. (3) The relationship is also so intense that it may tend to activate sexual and other improprieties.

Such features combine to distinguish the therapeutic relationship in psychiatry (and perhaps in the mental health field more generally) from the doctor–patient relationship in most other branches of medicine. For example, the relationship or alliance between psychiatrist and patient is believed by many

---

[6] These concerns over the principle of autonomy rest on fundamental and contrary assumptions and value, some more liberal, others more paternalistic. For a fuller discussion of such issues see Dunn (1998) and Radden (2003).

to be the central causal factor in the healing process. This relationship, it has been said, is not only a necessary but "perhaps often [a] *sufficient condition* for improvement in any kind of psychotherapy" (Frank and Frank 1991: 40, our emphasis). Granted, the doctor–patient relationship is recognized to be an important ingredient in many other branches of medicine; but in few others could the relationship be said to be necessary and sufficient for healing. (The theoretical underpinnings of, and empirical support for, these claims are discussed more fully in Chapter 2.)

That psychiatry is a practice requiring a heightened ethical attention to interpersonal relationships due to this factor is a very generally accepted presumption. One aspect of interpersonal relationships that has received considerable acknowledgment in psychiatry is the notion of professional "boundaries" and "boundary violations" (Gabbard 1999; Gutheil and Gabbard 1998; Kroll 2001; Martinez 2000; Radden 2001; Simon 1992). And while there is no agreement over the details, it is widely held that such attention can be successfully captured and codified in the discourse employing the metaphor of "boundaries." Codes of behavior have been elaborated that impose precise restrictions on the psychiatrist's comportment, personal expression, communication, and actions in every aspect of his dealings with his patient. Explaining the rationale for such rules, Glen Gabbard has noted that such boundaries "are structural characteristics of the relationship that allow the therapist to interact with warmth, empathy, and spontaneity within certain conditions that create a climate of safety. One might say that the external boundaries of the treatment are established so that the psychological boundaries between patient and therapist can be crossed through a number of means that are common to psychotherapeutic experience. These would include identification, empathy, projection, introjection, and projective identification" (Gabbard 1999: 143).

Restrictions such as these are maintained with the explicit goal of delimiting these boundaries—and the implicit admission that looser behavior is permissible in the practice of other areas of medicine. In no other medical specialty is the practitioner's conduct subjected to this degree of scrutiny and monitoring, and no other medical specialties have addressed such concerns as extensively and in so much detail.

Gabbard emphasizes that "external boundaries" must be established and maintained in order to safely permit the intense, interpersonal responses engendered by the setting. This dynamic is illustrated in the following case, where the practitioner must acknowledge and deal with his own feelings while at the same time refraining from crossing external, sexual boundaries.

Dr P is working with one of his first patients in the medication clinic, an attractive woman in her twenties who is a "dancer" in an upscale topless bar. She complains of depression and relationship problems with men and sees a psychologist for psychotherapy. She routinely comes to her medication clinic sessions wearing tight-fitting, seductive attire. The patient has a history of father–daughter incest, which she usually discusses in a flaunting, invulnerable fashion. Only recently, after 10 visits, does the patient begin to show signs of fragility and shame when relating a painful moment during her psychotherapy. Dr P has become aware of stirrings of desire for the patient with her newly revealed vulnerability. He is worried about what this means for him as a doctor and for the viability of his treatment relationship.

This case illustrates an additional feature that the *Annotations* also emphasize—the distinctiveness of the issues raised within psychiatric treatment. Almost invariably, it is noted, "sensitive and private" information is dealt with, demanding an especially high standard of confidentiality on the part of the psychiatrist. (See also Wahl 1999.)

These sensitive and private aspects of the material dealt with in psychiatric practice impose extra ethical constraints on practitioners in two separate ways. First, the strong natural impulse toward privacy is widely privileged in our society, and patients are entitled to have their confidences respected, if only as a protection against feelings of exposure, embarrassment, and shame. Second, the patient's fears over privacy are well founded because of the negative effects of such disclosures. Negative associations and consequent stigma still attach to the category of mental disorder. Indeed, it is stigma that is without parallel in the class of nonpsychiatric disorders. (Taken individually, certain conditions such as AIDS have specific associations that are comparable, needless to say.) Such stigma and negative attitudes result in fear and rejection of afflicted patients as well as overt and covert discrimination in the employment and insurance arenas. Extreme confidentiality is required to protect the patient from negative societal attitudes and resultant discriminatory and exclusionary behavior.

Consider the stakes faced by a husband and wife in the following case example:

Frederick W was persuaded to come to the Psychiatric Emergency Service after his wife found him drunk, sitting in the bathtub at

home, fully dressed, and with a pistol in his hand. Mr. W chairs
the board of a local corporation, the headquarters of which are
the economic center of this moderate-sized town. Mrs. W has been
terrified and ashamed about the entire process to date: finding her
husband in such desperate straits, having to disarm him and bring
him to the hospital, waiting for hours for him to sober up, and now,
perhaps worst of all, facing the possibility that he will be hospitalized in the "psych ward" and she will have to address his where-
abouts with family, friends, and business partners. She appears to
the emergency staff to be more concerned with who knows about
her husband's state than what care should be provided to him.

Mr. and Mrs. W must deal with issues that go well beyond the immediate medical ones imposed by Mr. W's inebriated condition. The interest
this couple has in the practitioner's promise of confidentiality is enormous,
deriving as it does from the potential stigma, from the self-imposed stigma
of shame and humiliation; as well as from the real risk of discriminatory
consequences. Both understood as part of a discussion of preserving the
frame or boundary of the therapeutic relationship, and treated as a separate
ethical concern, the issue of confidentiality has been recognized to be of
the greatest significance for psychiatric ethics. Its link with stigma and discrimination has been consistently emphasized. Less stressed, however, has
been the equally telling point made in the *Annotations*: the material dealt
with in therapy, not always, of course, but typically, is by its nature especially
private and sensitive. And again, although greater harm may be wrought by
breaches of confidentiality in relation to particular, sensitive diagnoses in the
rest of medicine, nonpsychiatric disorders taken as a group are not as vulnerable as mental disorders to the consequences of such breaches.

Psychiatric Diagnosis as Science

While Thomas Szasz's book, *The Myth of Mental Illness,* is well known to
the educated public, neurosurgery has no book entitled "The Myth of Brain
Tumors" (David Waller M.D., personal communication, 1997).

A set of persistent ethical issues with few or no parallels in the rest of
medicine concerns psychiatric diagnosis. The nature of psychiatric disorder, its epistemological status, and the social and psychological effects of

diagnosis, have long been the focus of psychiatric ethics and remain so today (Horwitz 2002; Poland et al. 1994; Reich 1999; Sadler 2002, 2003, 2004, 2005; Sadler et al. 1994; Szasz 1974). Other areas of medicine have at times given rise to somewhat similar ethical concerns over diagnosis. There have been debates over the disorder status of pregnancy, for example, and over the psychosomatic origins of certain conditions such as fibromyalgia or chronic Lyme disease. But nowhere else throughout the rest of medicine can be found such sustained focus on the ethics of diagnosis.

The popular suspicion that diagnostic categories reflect less a taxonomy of biologically based deficits or dysfunctions of the brain than arbitrary social constructions continues to challenge and subvert the tenets of biological psychiatry. This view finds support in a past history of misuses of diagnosis, most glaring in the former Soviet Union (Bloch and Chodoff 1981; Bloch et al. 1999; Fulford et al. 1993). Nearer to home, it points to the use of psychiatric diagnosis to affirm exclusionary social norms: misogyny and homophobia, for example, in diagnostic categories such as masochistic personality disorder (Caplan 1992, 1995a, 1995b; Caplan and Gans 1991) and homosexuality (Bayer 1981; Sadler 2005). Because major disorders of psychiatry have as yet no known biological causes, those skeptical of the scientific status or of the social meaning and effects of psychiatric diagnosis have emphasized its witting or unwitting power, and its potential for abuse.

Not only including but also going beyond these issues associated with diagnosis and diagnostic classification is the controversy attaching to much of the theory, knowledge base, and practice, of psychiatry, even today. In exploring psychiatry's status as a bioethical "ugly duckling," Bill Fulford and Tony Hope contrasted the way values are embedded in physical illness concepts with the way values in mental illness concepts remain unsettled and unresolved (Fulford and Hope 1994). There are still deep disagreements over such fundamentals as what sort of thing mental illness is, and how to understand it, they emphasized. Mental illness, as they put it, "differs from physical illness (overall) precisely in that our values are less widely shared— the criteria by which we judge mental conditions to be good or bad being open and problematic where the corresponding criteria for physical conditions are (relatively) closed and unproblematic" (Fulford and Hope 1994: 693). More recently Donna Dickenson and Fulford have developed related ideas by showing that compared with cases in the rest of medicine, cases from psychiatric practice routinely implicate deep philosophical questions of metaphysics, epistemology, and the philosophy of science, as well as ethics, in ways that inextricably tie psychiatry to philosophical assumptions and ideas. Owing to these features, psychiatric practice cannot easily be subsumed under the standard model of biomedical ethics, where medicine's primary values are largely agreed-upon and noncontroversial (Dickenson and Fulford 2000; Fulford 2004).

Conclusion

The three substantive ethical issues introduced here—difficulties applying the concept of autonomy to psychiatric patients, the ethical niceties around "boundaries," and ethical implications of psychiatric diagnosis—reflect some of the most obvious instances where psychiatry differs from other medical practice. These, and some other issues apparently distinctive to psychiatry or at the least magnified by the mental health care setting, have received considerable attention by those in psychiatry and in philosophy. But except in the *Annotations*, the extent to which these arise out of features distinguishing psychiatric practice has rarely been stressed. It is often implied, for example, that the aspects of ethically challenging cases from psychiatry differ no more from those found in internal medicine, geriatrics, or surgery than those do from one another. And the commonalities, which are legion, have received more attention than the differences.

In the next chapter, we try to make good that failure of emphasis with a more systematic review of the features of the social and medical practice of psychiatry that serve to separate it from other medical subspecialties and that call for unique ethical responses. These features will also help resolve the question, introduced earlier, of the applicability of the consumer model. They will show, we believe, that the consumer model is sometimes inappropriately extended to the psychiatric setting and that in the case of severe mental disorder, it is often applicable during only part of the patient's experience of disorder.

To the extent that the consumer model is appropriate, ethical demands on psychiatric practice will be more easily derived from the generic principles of biomedical ethics. To the extent that it is not, they will require something that goes above and beyond those principles. But to presume that the consumer model is always applicable to the psychiatric setting, as many do today, and to adopt an ethical framework based on that presumption before carefully examining and acknowledging not only the similarities but also the differences between psychiatric practice and other areas of medicine is, we believe, to put the cart before the horse. In the following chapter, these differences will receive the attention they deserve.

2 The Distinctiveness of the Psychiatric Setting

Introduction

Most previous analyses have dwelt on one or another particular feature of the setting including, as we saw, concerns over patient autonomy, boundary issues, and psychiatric diagnosis. And each of these features, taken alone, has been recognized to impose special ethical demands on practitioners, it is true. Still, we believe that discussions heretofore for the most part understated the distinctness of psychiatric practice or ignored the ethical significance of that distinctness, or both.

In this chapter we continue the enumeration and explanation of the features of the psychiatry setting that, in combination, serve to distinguish it from others. Some of these aspects of practice, noted by other researchers, have been introduced already; others are so obvious that their significance and implications have largely gone unremarked. Our claim, we emphasize again, is not that these characteristics separately distinguish psychiatry practice, but that taken together, this set of elements constitutes psychiatry as a distinctive practice. Overall, our purpose is to complete the demonstration, begun in Chapter 1, of why psychiatry requires more than biomedical ethics. In Chapters 3–7 we explain what sort of additional ethic and ethical framework that could be.

The features of psychiatric care that combine to make it a unique social practice are manifold, and are unevenly displayed across the different settings and types of psychiatric practice.[1] The culture of psychiatry and psychiatric care is a complex, heterogeneous, fast changing, and contradictory one, which defies easy summary, as T. M. Luhrmann demonstrated in her valuable anthropological survey of the state of the profession in the last decades of the twentieth century (Luhrmann 2000).

Much the same can be said of the population receiving mental health care in that setting. In addition to patients incapacitated by their disorder, psychiatrists also see those effectively treated and responding unexceptionally to social and occupational challenges in everyday life; moreover, they care for every imaginable case between these two extremes. Our attention here, we want again to emphasize, is directed toward the setting where patients are treated for major mental disorders such as schizophrenia, depression, bipolar disorder, and obsessive compulsive disorder.

Features of the culture of psychiatrists, patients, and their care will be the focus of this chapter, including aspects of the patients themselves, their disorders, the historical and cultural context in which, and societal structures through which, psychiatric practice is undertaken, and aspects of psychiatric lore and practice. The composite of these different features will be referred to in what follows as the "psychiatry setting." Although these are somewhat artificial divisions, we have sorted the features of the psychiatry setting into eight categories: (i) patient vulnerabilities; (ii) patient attitudes toward symptoms; (iii) psychiatric disorders as long-term disorders; (iv) societal structures; (v) stigma and controversy over mental disorder, and (vi) aspects of the therapeutic project. Two more recent changes affecting the psychiatry setting, (vii) managed care delivery systems and (viii) today's consumer movements, and their ethical implications, are then noted.

Patient Vulnerabilities

If only temporarily and partially, severely ill psychiatric patients are often deprived of the capabilities required for an exercise of autonomy and of their best defenses against exploitation: their judgment in matters concerning their

---

[1] These generalizations about psychiatric practice are entirely drawn from, and likely limited to, the North American culture of the late-twentieth and early-twenty-first centuries.

immediate and long-term self-interest; their reasoning ability, their insight into their own condition, their self-control, their personal and psychic integration, their capacity to communicate their concerns and needs to others, and their perceptions of other people's responses. Almost all writing about mental illness emphasizes this aspect of its effect on patients. By virtue of their emotional distress and dysfunction, it has been estimated, mentally ill people are "among the most vulnerable of any group" (Bloch and Pargiter 1999: 101).

Three important disclaimers apply immediately, however. First, this assessment in no way detracts from the courage, persistence, ingenuity, and frequent effectiveness shown by psychiatric patients as they live, do battle with, and effectively "manage" their symptoms. Second, these incapacities are rarely total, permanent, or unremitting. Contrary to the gloomy prognoses that used to attach to most severe disorders (schizophrenia, in particular), long-term outcome studies suggest that a significant number of those who suffer such disorders recover completely or with only mild impairment (Davidson and McGlashan 1997; Thomas 1997; Topor 2001). And finally, as recent research suggests, these incapacities may be in some part an artifact of stigma, negative social attitudes, and diminished expectations, rather than symptoms of the disorder (Barham 1997; Davidson 2003). They could be remedied, or at least reduced, merely through a transformation of social attitudes.

All that said, we maintain that at least at certain times, these obstacles to autonomous functioning are an aspect of many mental patients' lives and experience and as such they call for certain moral responses from, and require certain types of character in, practitioners.

As well as providing practitioners with moral reasons to respond and act in particular ways, these patient vulnerabilities require attention because they affect parts of the person—cognitive, affective, communicative, and volitional capabilities—that have been linked with traditional conceptions of personhood, agency, self, and self-identity. Paul McHugh and Phillip Slavney discuss the "ontological assault" bodily illness has been said to make on a person. This may be an appropriate way of depicting many illnesses, they observe, but "it will not do for psychiatric illness. In psychiatric illness, the ontological assault is not on the body but *on the self* ... the primary abnormality in psychiatric disorders is an alteration in the patient's thinking, mood, or behavior and ... these phenomena are more closely tied to his sense of self, to his essence as a person, to his existential being than are coughs, rashes, deformities, or pains" (McHugh and Slavney 1987: 95–96, emphasis added).

Others have made similar or related observations. In his 2003 Tanner Lectures Jonathan Glover spoke of what he called the cluster of values to do with identity; this cluster, he remarked "has a more problematic relation to psychiatric disorders, because some of those disorders can change the central core of a person" (Glover 2003: 05). Explaining the fear and consequent stigma associated with severe mental disorder, James Lindemann Nelson sketched the link with personhood this way: to be—or to have been—mentally ill "is still seen ... as defective in those features of cognition or agency that we tend to prize as distinctive to and definitive of human personhood" (Nelson 2003: 01). Luhrmann ties personhood and self-identity to the attitudes in others prompted by mental illness. We are terrified by psychosis and depression, she insists, because mental illness "distorts the defining features of personhood." These aspects of madness separate it from other diseases, and those who are mad are different: "Their illnesses are part of *who they are* in a way that seems different from the alien invasion of a cancer" (Luhrmann 2000: 270–271, our emphasis).

These are large claims. What's more, they differ: some allude to the self or person in metaphysical terms, others make psychological claims about the way in which the subject perceives or knows herself. Theories of self-identity vary in the extent to which they imply that an individual's psychological attributes all form part of "who they are," for example. A "narrative self" theory portrays the "author" of the self-narrative as—with others—selecting the features that comport with a story she constructs, rather than the passive recipient of the life experiences she has been dealt (Nelson 2001; Schechtman 1996). On such an analysis, a person's professional or familial role, or ongoing physical disease, may be more central to her identity than an isolated episode of mental disorder. So the extent that disorder affects the individual self-identity of patients may depend on the self-identity, as well as perhaps the theory of self-identity, involved.

McHugh and Slavney, Glover, Nelson, and Luhrmann are at least right in supposing that mental disorder compromises the capabilities often associated with agency, self, and self-identity, and so that disorder seems to jeopardize traits we value, and to threaten moral categories forming our understanding of our humanity and personhood. This will readily explain others' attitudes and some of the attendant stigma and fear engendered by mental disorder, as Luhrmann points out. Given what we know of internalized stigma, it may well result in a negative self-identity, as well (Davidson 2003). Unlike some theorists today, we do not reject the metaphysical conception of self presupposed in the claims just made linking personhood to the traits often affected by mental disorder. But nor do we defend it here. The metaphysical question is controversial: many would deny the existence of an essence of personhood such as McHugh and Slavney presuppose. Mistaken or not, however, this way of attributing selfhood remains widespread in our culture. To the extent that it continues to form many a self-conception, the associations with personhood will have powerful implications that cannot easily be ignored.

One such implication, then, is that psychiatric disorder magnifies the patient's vulnerability through its effect on the attributes associated (misguidedly or not) with personhood. Psychiatric disorder adds to that vulnerability in a second important way, moreover: it often compromises basic communicative capabilities. Other medical conditions, and indeed, communicative disabilities themselves, such as deafness, also interfere with these capabilities. But the ability to get care through a communication of symptoms is especially vital with mental disorders because these disorders so often lack reliable bodily or behavioral indicators. As the sole basis for diagnosis in many instances, and the decisive one in others, the psychiatric patient's communicated symptoms possess unusual significance. Unconsciousness, or aphasia, might well rob a person of communicative capabilities more surely and totally than schizophrenia or depression. With schizophrenia or depression, though, because observers as yet possess few clues to independently ascertain what is going on and how to proceed, problems communicating symptoms have added—often crucial—importance.

Not all psychiatric patients exhibit incapacities such as these, and psychiatric patients are rarely, if ever, wanting in all of these ways. Nor are they the only group with such disadvantages. The organic dementias and injuries to the brain also deprive their sufferers of the capabilities enumerated above, for example, as, more consistently, do developmental and learning disorders of childhood, and cognitive delay. And indeed, some vulnerability to exploitation, dependence, and inherent inequality, it has even been said, characterizes a client in any professional relationship (Pellegrino and Thomasma 1993).

The portrait of mental patients that emphasizes their vulnerability has become controversial in contemporary times. The mental health consumers (service users, survivors, mad pride, and recovery) groups introduced in Chapter 1, together with political attempts to include mental disorder within the broader disabilities movement, all resist the totalizing, essentializing, and negative stereotyping invited by an overemphasis on the deficiencies enumerated above.

The emergence of these movements is a critical development, with far-reaching implications for psychiatric ethics; we will need to return to it throughout the following chapters. These new voices, in some ways uniquely placed to speak on the matter of how they are to be understood, must be heard and heeded. But, although we recognize the following claim will always need qualification in the particular case—not only in application to a particular practice setting and a given patient but also to the stage in the patient's illness experience—the analysis that follows suggests that compared to adult patients and clients in many other professional settings, psychiatric patients are often notably disadvantaged and rendered singularly vulnerable by their symptoms and the nature of their disorder.

Some of the implications of these vulnerabilities for psychiatric ethics are fairly obvious. Whatever the degree of these patients' proneness to neglect, exploitation, abuse, and to the harms of violated confidentiality, this vulnerability will apparently place an extra ethical burden on those who care for such patients, as well as those interacting with them in a research setting. It will call, we might put it, for added virtues, or added virtue, in practitioners.

This straightforward and obvious point about the moral demands imposed by patients' vulnerabilities may perhaps have been made without invoking the idea of virtues, we concede, although not as effectively. It might have been said that such vulnerability calls for extra duties on the part of the practitioner. But with many virtue ethicists today, we believe in an approach that deems such duties to be derivative: drawn from the traits of the virtuous person. And in the present volume the point is expressed in terms of the demands the patients' vulnerabilities impose on the character of the practitioner, and of the additional virtue or virtues called for. (Which virtues these are, and exactly how they are to be acquired and cultivated, will be explored in subsequent chapters.)

Many in today's consumer movements merely ask to be recognized as whole individuals with assets and imperfections like the rest of us, requesting that they be regarded, and treated, as persons rather than "cases." But other claims are more radical. In an effort to emphasize positive traits and strengths, rather than weaknesses and vulnerabilities, and thus to "valorize" mental disorder, some have rejected not only the language but also the traditional roles of mental health care. Rather than a healer, the practitioner is cast in the role of something closer to an advisor, coach, or collaborator than a doctor—an assistant in achieving one's self-defined life goals. This will likely pose dilemmas for the practitioner, as she negotiates between her own conception of her role and the conception assumed, adopted, or even urged, by the patient. One such challenge is illustrated below: the practitioner, Dr. M encounters a dilemma of what might be termed "political negotiation."

> The parents of a 17-year-old undergoing treatment for Dysthymia had called Dr. M along with Dr. B. The patient entered the office, under his arm a well-thumbed copy of Foucault's *Madness and Civilization*. "What seems to be going on?," asked Dr. M. "You tell me," responded the patient, smirking: "My mom figures Dr. B needs a second opinion. . . I guess he isn't sure what he's doing." Dr. M suggested the patient tell her about his treatment with Dr B. His response: "It's all bullshit. I feel fine, I AM fine. It's Dr. B who's messed up, man."

Dr. M's fundamental professional responsibility here is to interview the patient and provide an assessment of his condition. Yet in order to do so, she may be required to refrain from challenging the patient's assumptions about his symptoms, with which she is in complete disagreement, and may even need to appear to accept his characterization of her colleague Dr. B.

Political negotiation dilemmas for practitioners such as this one will sometimes even include forging an alliance with the patient that denies or sidesteps its characterization as therapeutic. More generally, it will require greater tact, empathy, and integrity than would be required in doctor–patient relationships that unequivocally accord the practitioner the customary function as healer, and therefore enjoy a shared and stable understanding of each participant's role.

Subjective Attitudes toward Symptoms

The nature of some psychiatric symptoms provides a further reason to distinguish these from most other medical conditions. Several mental disorders bring positive, gratifying, and even desirable experiences for patients. Examples include the increased and socially rewarding energy of mania, the pleasing grandiosity of narcissism, and the euphoric intoxication of addiction.

In addition, the presumption that (at least in the face of medical opinion) those experiencing symptoms will usually acknowledge that such symptoms indicate disorder—while at least usually true of other medical symptoms—is not as consistently true for psychiatric symptoms. It is common for patients to deny or fail to recognize their experiences or behavior as symptoms of a disorder—and to undergo changes in these attitudes toward their symptoms as a manifestation of the disorder itself. Such differences engender further communicative difficulties. Attitudes toward ordinary medical symptoms bring customary expectations and responses from those hearing the complaint, including sympathy and a willingness to help. And these expectations and patterns of response make up what is usually an integrated, smooth, and relatively easy communicative exchange. The difference in attitudes and expectations accompanying psychiatric symptoms serve to disrupt and interfere with such communicative engagement. Without an exceptionally strong doctor–patient alliance, such complex and ambivalent attitudes on the part of patients would go unchecked and likely undermine, or even prevent, effective treatment.

The following example illustrates some of the complexity inherent in maintaining the alliance with a patient exhibiting such ambivalence vis à vis his symptoms.

> After treatment with a potent monoamine oxidase inhibitor, a
> depressed postal clerk has "switched" from depression to mania,
> over the course of a day or two. He presents to the clinician with
> a packed briefcase full of notes and briefs. He says: "Thank you
> Doctor, for making me feel so good … let me tell you the plans I
> have for a restructuring of General Motors … I have made several
> calls to Lee Iacocca to share these plans, but he hasn't returned my
> calls … perhaps I shouldn't have called at 3 am this morning."

The clinician must not only deal with the grandiose beliefs of his patient here. He must also negotiate through a redefinition of the patient's experience as ill, and convince him to accept additional treatment. Finally, he must help the patient recognize the validity of each person's role, the practitioner's as expert healer, and the role of himself as patient.

Psychiatric Patients as Long-Term Patients

Serious mental disorders such as schizophrenia, bipolar disorder, recurrent or chronic major depression, and obsessive-compulsive disorder are very often long-term disorders.[2] Some will remit, others will not, but medical knowledge leaves the question of outcome in considerable doubt for most people suffering major mental disorders such as these, and temporary remission remains linked with at least possible, and often probable, recurrence.

As today's recovery movement emphasizes, permanent recovery does occur, and everyone with mental disorder, even with these severe mental disorders, has reason for hope (Barham 1997; Bracken and Thomas 2005; Davidson and McGlashan 1997; Neugeboren 1999; Whitaker 2002). Nonetheless, lack of knowledge about mental disorders requires us to see the notion of a long-term patient, in two distinct ways. Not only are "long-term patients" those requiring years of treatment; in addition, long-term patients include those who may relapse even when, due to an amelioration in their condition, they leave the psychiatric setting. In the psychiatry setting, patients are often long-term patients in both senses.

This characteristic of the psychiatric setting imposes special ethical demands on the practitioner. When some unidentified—and presently unidentifiable—subgroup of patients will prove to suffer a recurrence of disorder, the practitioner's moral and ethical situation, including the alliance formed with every patient, will be relatively more serious, burdensome, and complex.[3]

At least two discussions acknowledge this long-term nature of many psychiatric patients, the first in the literature on the boundaries of the therapeutic relationship. Because the future is uncertain, and might see the resumption of a therapeutic relationship long ago terminated, more stringent rules and constraints to govern every nuance of doctor–patient relationships are

---

[2] This is not true of every disorder seen in a psychiatric setting, of course. For example, psychiatrists also see patients with life transition issues, wayward children, and marital complaints.

[3] This feature of psychiatric illness may have theoretical implications for attempts to analogize the doctor–patient relationship with that of friendship. (See, for example, Illingworth 1988; Oakley and Cocking 2001; Veatch 1991.) Oakley and Cocking contrast the terminating or governing conditions between these two sorts of relationship: a doctor is disposed to end relationships with patients *when there was no longer need for medical care*, yet "it is not part of the nature of the norms of friendship that the relationship ... should cease simply because . . . [care] is no longer needed by one's friend" (Oakley and Cocking 2001: 52). The long-term nature of patients in mental health care makes it something of an anomalous case, on this dichotomy, and in certain ways farther from many usual doctor–patient relationships and closer to friendship.

widely believed necessary, including rules forbidding any present or future sexual contact with patients. As those arguing for the maintenance of strict boundaries in all psychiatric practice have pointed out, patients commonly recontact the therapist for further consultation or treatment in the years following the end of formal treatment (Gabbard 1999: 149).

There is a second ethical implication of the long-term aspect of much mental disorder. This one ties to the observation, made earlier, that psychiatric disorders affect traits and capabilities allied to personhood and often to self-identity. Long-term traits, including the symptoms of any severe mental disorder, will more likely become part of a person's self-identity than will those of shorter duration. Although most evidently true of those suffering personality disorders, because they are a set of long-term characteristic and defining traits, this will also be true of other conditions. Even on a narrative analysis, which as we saw grants a power of selection to the author of the self-narrative, a decade of depression symptoms can hardly fail to form part, if only part, of a person's story and self-identity.

Societal Structures

Legal and policy responses to the perceived disadvantages and vulnerabilities often attributable to psychiatric patients have included certain protections and restrictions. The criminal law procedures around fitness to stand trial and the defense of criminal insanity are examples of these. Other examples include statutes permitting involuntary treatment and involuntary confinement—laws that, as we saw earlier, place the psychiatrist in a distinctive ethical position. Similarly, in the research setting, we find acknowledgment that patients with some mental disorders will be particularly vulnerable to exploitation by researchers.[4] (Historically, attitudes toward mental disorder have consistently portrayed the mentally ill as incompetent, irrational, and entirely lacking the capabilities required for autonomy. So the extent to which policy responses such as these accord with patients' actual capabilities is, as we saw earlier, controversial and contested.)

The part played by psychiatrists in these legal and public policy roles carries several additional implications for the moral psychology and character

---

[4] See for example, a recent report by the National Bioethics Advisory Commission, (NBAC 1998), or Elliott's discussion of depression and competence in research (Elliott 1999: Chapter 5); nonetheless, this concern can also be overstated. For a counterbalancing generalization, see Roberts and Roberts (1999).

of the psychiatrist. First, psychiatrists are required to be agents of the state. They must often act as protector of the public as well as healer, not only caring for the patient but also ensuring community safety. Specific mental health legislation sets psychiatry apart from the rest of medicine, as Allen Fraser has noted, because such legislation contains "a tension between legally requiring reluctant patients to accept treatment in their best interests, and treatment or detention for the benefit of others." (In pointing out that the psychiatrist, "has an obligation to the family of his patients, and also to members of society" (Fraser 2000), Fraser contrasts the psychiatrist with other doctors. This overstates the case: sometimes other doctors undertake these obligations too. The important point is that psychiatrists are unfailingly expected to do so.) Undertaking these two, distinct, directives, likely often in tension, will call for a degree of integrity and moral imagination not usually demanded of the medical practitioner. Perhaps, as Fraser suggests, only the development of moral virtues will protect the psychiatrist from the potentially corrupting power entailed in this unique societal responsibility.

There is an additional point, which we develop more fully in later chapters. Charged with the power of civil commitment, the psychiatrist may also be expected to go above and beyond the ethical demands of the immediate situation by avoiding even the public appearance of unethical conduct as well as avoiding any actual unethical conduct. This higher standard, sometimes expected of figures in government office, calls for psychiatrists to conduct themselves in such a way as to avoid even the suggestion of impropriety, the hint of self-interest, or whiff of exploitative motives. These unique powers, we demonstrate, call for the appearance, as well as the reality, of virtue.

The social role nowadays accorded practitioners in psychiatry may well change in the years to come. Certainly, much of the emphasis of the political struggles of today's consumer movements has been on laws and policies around coerced treatment and seclusion. And Patrick Bracken and Philip Thomas in their proposals for what they entitle "postpsychiatry," foresee a world where mental health policy has relinquished the coercive trappings of "modernist" approaches to mental disorder and entirely eliminated such roles. As they put it, "if genuine trust is ever to be established between the medical profession and those who suffer episodes of madness, there needs to be a substantial weakening of the link between treatment and coercion." This is not to say that society should never remove a person's liberty on account of mental disorder, but the authority today accorded to medical psychiatry should be replaced with increased "lay involvement," which they explain as voluntary sector organizations and self-help groups, and with the use of advanced care directives (Bracken and Thomas 2005: 12).

If these apparently utopian goals can one day be met then, undoubtedly, the distinctive ethical demands on practitioners associated with these social roles in present-day psychiatry will alter, and perhaps wane. Until that time, however, we maintain that special moral demands are called for in the character of practitioners.

Stigma and Controversy over Mental Disorder

The social stigma surrounding mental disorder since ancient times has led to exclusion, abuse, and prejudice through to the present day (Dain 1999; Fabrega 1990, 1991; Sedgwick 1982). The extent to which modern day medical psychiatry, and more enlightened public policy, have together succeeded in unseating these social attitudes—or have at most replaced them with comparably damaging and negative stereotypes—is disputed by scholars and historians of medicine. Michel Foucault, for example, insists that modern medicine has "silenced" the mentally ill, extinguishing their very humanity (Foucault 1971). Other analyses paint a quite different picture, and suggest that modern psychiatry is to be credited with transforming the lives of those suffering such afflictions (Shorter 1997; U.S. Surgeon General 1999).

These controversies and alternative readings of the changes wrought through the last century and a half of institutionalized psychiatry are difficult to evaluate. What we can be sure of is that although the religious and moralistic prejudices that used to attach to madness may be for the most part forgotten in today's Westernized cultures, such cultures still cleave—for better or worse—to the traditional Western ideals noted earlier. They value the capabilities on which agency, personhood, and self-identity depend; they also prefer independence over dependence, rationality over illogic, communicative transparency over unintelligibility, self-control over impulsiveness, agency over passivity, and unity of the psyche over its fracture and disintegration. Only if we acknowledge this can we recognize how deep and intransigent are the roots of stigma over mental disorder.

The political philosopher Nancy Fraser (and others) have spoken of two distinct and irreducible paradigms of justice. The more familiar of these is the redistributive one associated with economic justice. The other is a "recognition" paradigm that requires the elimination of injustices rooted in cultural patterns of representation, communication, and interpretation (Fraser 2003).

Injustices remedied by the distribution paradigm are those such as exploitation, economic marginalization, and deprivation. The recognition paradigm remedies cultural injustices (Fraser 2003: 6). Fraser applies the recognition paradigm to four different collective identities: those based on class, gender, race, and "despised sexualities." But her analysis will arguably apply to other groups as well, including the collective identity of the mentally ill. Acknowledging this second paradigm, we can see that Western cultures such as ours have barely begun to contend with the stigma that attaches to mental disorder.

An explanation of the persistence with which negative associations attach to psychiatric disorder has also been sought in the ignorance that attaches to these disorders—ignorance over their causes, course, and cure. Describing the many stereotypes that have signified madness in the visual arts, Sander Gilman remarks that such stereotyping is "the product of the application of existing paradigms to those aspects of the universe which a culture has defined as *inherently inexplicable"* (Gilman 1982: Preface i, our emphasis). Even today, such "root metaphors" affect and curtail our perception of mental disorder and its sufferers, Gilman believes. If mental disorder were understood as well as are most other medical conditions then, it might be supposed, this tie to its present, negative associations would loosen.

Those practicing psychiatry today frequently subscribe, completely or in part, to a medical model. The application to psychiatry of the medical model has been seen as fitting by its supporters because of what is conceived to be the completeness of the parallel between "mental" and other medical disorders.[5] The medical model has also been endorsed because, it is believed, its application to psychiatric disorders should serve to de-mystify them. Certainly we hope medical science will eventually come to identify and explain states of mental disorder with reference to specific biological markers, thus eliminating some aspects of the obscurity and fear presently surrounding them. Yet until mental disorder is eliminated entirely, the above reasoning suggests, some of its negative associations will likely persist. A biomedical explanation of mental illness alone may not eliminate stigma. Rooted in the fear and incomprehension of other people, such attitudes can persist in the face of well-explained odd behavior, novel cultural customs, and indeed cultural transitions. Some surmise that stigma is borne of cultural distrust of alterity or "otherness," and if so, linked to the social process

[5] For a thoughtful and carefully reasoned challenge to the presuppositions underlying this position, see Pickering (2006).

of determining deviance as such, it will be ineluctably wedded to the social aspects of mental illness (Gaines 1992; Sadler 2005).

Whatever their source, it is undoubtedly true that as long as the present negative associations of mental disorder survive, psychiatric patients will remain at increased risk of prejudicial and discriminatory treatment, exploitation, and the damaging social attitudes that in turn give rise to internalized stigma. Only its extent may be challenged. And for this reason as well we believe the deep-seated vulnerability of psychiatric patients calls for a greater attention to ethical behavior in psychiatrists than would be required of those engaged in many other forms of medical practice.

The controversy surrounding mental disorder also adds to the risk of prejudicial treatment for its sufferers. The disagreements, noted in Chapter 1, are legion: what mental disorder is, indeed whether it exists; how it should be explained and how treated; whether it is usefully characterized in mentalistic terms at all; the extent of its status as a social construction; the relationship it bears to other forms of human suffering; the question of who are the experts on mental disorder (sufferers or practitioners) and what kind of knowledge is required; the question of what kind of treatment (if any), by whom, should be offered in response to it. These and other fundamental matters are continuing subjects of controversy and disagreement in our culture today, and debated not merely by theorists but at the broad societal level. Many of these questions were first raised as long ago as the 1950s–1970s. Yet general interest in them shows little sign of abating, and any hope of resolving them seems as vain as ever. Similar questions are from time to time raised in relation to be some other medical conditions, undoubtedly. Consider the conflicting attitudes around smoking, and obesity, for example, or around controversial treatments and their side effects. Yet the divisions are deeper with psychiatric disorders. The controversies are more profound, affecting not one or another condition but the broad category of mental disorder *tout court*. And the areas of disagreement seem to be more extensive.

Aspects of the Therapeutic Project

Two additional differences between the psychiatric setting and other medical practices, each providing additional moral reasons for the practitioner, can best be understood through an acknowledgment of aspects of the therapeutic project. First, the therapeutic project in the psychiatry setting is frequently, existentially, and morally momentous—changing aspects of the patient understood in notably holistic terms, involving traits associated with personhood. The moral significance of this project exposes the patient to additional dangers from exploitation and imposes an extra moral burden on the therapist. Second, the importance of the therapeutic alliance in psychiatry, believed a key ingredient in therapeutic effectiveness, calls for special ethical sensitivities and responses on the part of the practitioner.

The Project

In every field of medicine an approach treating the patient as a whole person—possessing a psyche as well as a body, and a lived life as well as a temporary ailment—is one strongly advocated, although not always practiced, today (Alderson 1991; Aronowitz 1998; Christie and Hoffmaster 1986; Holmes and Lindley 1989; Jackson 1999; Sherwin 1992). This holistic approach in psychiatry includes judging the patient as a psycho-socio-cultural whole, embedded in a social, relational, and meaning-giving nexus. In addition, it involves recognition of the patient as an identity across stretches of time—constituted as much by her past and future states as by her present ones. Thus the patient is associated less with particular actions as with more enduring states and dispositions—and with a life story. The patient is a human agent and a person in the richest philosophical sense, a socially and culturally embedded, psycho-physical whole, possessed of a self-narrative.

Regardless of the medical specialty involved, this holistic approach is increasingly prescribed, for any number of reasons. Yet here, too, psychiatry is somewhat different. There are additional and special reasons, distinctive to psychiatry, why the holistic approach is definitive of its particular focus and is not only ethically desirable, but close to unavoidable.

First, then, we want to emphasize that the holistic approach is called for, in the psychiatry setting, because of the nature of the project in psychiatry. Second, we want to show that such an approach is almost unavoidable in the practice of psychiatry and can be identified in the way the psychiatric project is understood and evaluated by practitioners, and in the way it is construed by patients. We believe this to be demonstrably true, although it has not always been acknowledged (and has even been explicitly denied).[6]

---

[6] See, for instance, Guze (1989).

The reasons why this holistic approach found in psychiatric treatment is ethically called for stem from the nature of the help sought, as well as the nature of the disorder suffered. The first of these were introduced earlier: the therapeutic project involves attributes associated with personhood. Psychiatry requires a holistic approach inasmuch as' it concerns itself with traits and states of the person culturally identified with personhood (and often with notions of self or "characterization" identity): not only inner states such as thoughts and beliefs, emotions, mood, attitudes, and motivations, as well as interpersonal relationships and communicative capacities, but also individuating aspects such as gender, race, and ethnicity. In contrast to fleeting qualities and passing ailments, any long-term attribute will likely shape the contours of the patient's self-identity and affect how others understand who the patient is. A second reason, then, is that psychiatric disorders are so often long-term disorders. Assertions as to the nature of personhood are metaphysical ones, and may perhaps be challenged at some theoretical level.[7] But the claim we make here is an empirical one, an observation about the philosophical ideas and ideals forming part of our culture's shared meanings. For better or worse, in our culture at least, the moral and metaphysical concept of personhood is allied to these traits.

The link between the states and traits that are disordered or diseased in psychiatric illness, and these fundamental capabilities constitutive of what—probably even biologically, certainly culturally, and we believe, metaphysically—makes us human persons, means the appropriate approach to the patient in the psychiatry setting is a holistic one. This holistic approach is actually employed in the practice setting; we want now to show, even if without complete acknowledgment. The framing of the goals of therapeutic intervention in psychiatry usually presupposes it; the subsequent evaluation of that intervention's success is so characterized, and finally, it is confirmed by patient accounts of the therapeutic encounter. (For an important

[7] That said, these assertions can avoid egregious forms of mind–body dualism. We do not need to accept a dualistic "ghost in the machine" account of the person to recognize that receiving medical care for diseased or aberrant thoughts, moods, attitudes, or desires is profoundly different from receiving medical care for almost all other medical ailments. These are embodied subjects, it is true. Yet human biology is such that conscious states—thoughts and feelings—are the locus of higher-level executive function. Similarly, troubles with judgment, perception, and communication are troubles with the means we have of maintaining our bodily integrity and physical well-being in the material and intersubjective world around us.

recent explication of the way the healing project in psychiatry is imbued with holism in these and other ways, see Ghaemi 2003.)

This claim is patently true of long-term psychotherapy, so we will focus our demonstration on two kinds of treatment where it is less immediately apparent, psychopharmacology and cognitive-behavioral approaches. First, even when adherence to a strictly biological model seems to reduce psychiatric practice to the dispensing of psychoactive drugs, diagnosis requires, and therapy is usually understood, in these same holistic terms. Very commonly, the patient wants help to feel better as a whole, and even such psychopharmacological intervention usually seeks to change permanent and pervasive states of being, traits, dispositions, and habits of mind, rather than precisely defined and narrow behavioral responses, or ideas. Successful long-term outcome in the seemingly straightforward response of a depressed patient to antidepressant medication, for example, depends on reorienting the patient to the meaning of the depressive event in his or her life, addressing the precipitants that caused the depressive event at this time in the life trajectory, and learning how to adjust so that the patient can adaptively deal with such precipitants in the future.

Moreover, although cognitive-behavioral treatment is explicitly oriented toward apparently limited goals, seeking outcomes in narrow, behaviorally defined terms, the effectiveness of such treatment is similarly evaluated in more holistic terms. Rather than evaluation using symptom checklists, healing is understood more globally—in terms of relapse prevention and improvements in life functioning. Indeed, fundamental assumptions about how the person relates to self, others, and the world, are explicitly addressed through the reform of the maladaptive assumed beliefs known as "schemata." Such schemata may be encompassing moral beliefs (e.g., "I hold myself to higher standards than others"); interpersonal beliefs ("People think I am insignificant"), even metaphysical beliefs ("the world is empty of meaning"). But they are in each case portrayed as broadly defined cognitive dispositions to respond (Erwin 2004).

Patients' own accounts of their care, whatever form their treatment took, provide a final confirmation that the therapeutic project requires these holistic terms (Barker et al. 1999; Custance 1952; Jamison 1995; Kaplan 1964; Kempe 1985; Slater 1998; Styron 1990; Read and Reynolds 1996). This is true throughout the long tradition of such memoirs, but it is increasingly so in our era of "identity politics," when self or personal identity have come to receive unparalleled attention. In some accounts, influenced by biological psychiatry, symptoms are depicted as the inconsequential effects of a diseased brain. But not infrequently, symptoms are depicted as meaningful aspects of experience and reality, and the goal of recovery is represented as one of integrating symptoms into a holistically understood self (Sadler 2007).[8] Even memoirs adopting a biomedical model emphasize the effects of the disorder on lived experience, and on self-identity. This is well illustrated in Simon Champ's memoir "A Most Precious Thread" (1999). Champ describes a "communication with himself" that allowed him to overcome the initial sense of disintegration accompanying the onset of his disorder, and gave him, he reports, "the most precious thread, a thread that has linked my evolving sense of self, a thread of self reclamation, a thread of movement toward a whole and integrated sense of self, away from the early fragmentation and confusion" (Champ 1999: 12).

Enhanced through "identity politics," the importance of cultural categories such as gender, race, and ethnicity to a person's self or characterization identity, deserves special attention here. The following case illustrates the centrality of gender identity and also the inescapably holistic terms in which that project is construed.

> John Nelson was a 17-year-old referred by his pediatrician and his parents. On the first visit, John explained why he was appointed to see an adolescent psychiatrist:
> "My parents sent me here because they're worried that I'm gay or something. All my friends are girls, I like to do "girly" things, I hate sports, I'd wear their clothes if I could get away with it. I can't wait until I grow up so I can become a woman. Until then, everyone, including my parents, make my life miserable. It's not fair, because I'm a good student and a good kid. I don't hurt anyone. Everyone except my real friends thinks I should be macho or something. My parents just want you to convert me into a macho boy. I'm not a macho boy. I'm me, and I just want to be accepted for the way I am. Why can't society just accept me?"

The way in which a gender sensitive practitioner will respond to such cases is explored at length in a later chapter (Chapter 4). Here, it is sufficient to note that this patient's whole self, person, and identity are the focus of his parents' concern, and—although he sees it differently from them—his own.

---

[8] For a fuller discussion of such memoirs see Radden (2008).

At its most ambitious then, we are looking at a deeply significant project, that of healing and reforming traits central to the patient's personhood. With respect to moral seriousness, this "existential audacity" of the therapeutic project is matched by few tasks undertaken in our culture except for the raising of children. Such ambitions add immeasurably to the patient's vulnerability and to the responsibility imposed on the psychiatrist.

The Alliance

Again in striking contrast to much, though not all, of the rest of medical practice, the self or *persona* of the practitioner is widely portrayed as entering into the therapeutic engagement in a particularly critical way because of the heightened importance of the therapeutic alliance between practitioner and patient. This point is emphasized in the APA *Annotations* (introduced in the Chapter 1). The relationship between doctor and patient is so "vital" a factor in effective treatment of the patient, as the *Annotations* put it, that preservation of optimal conditions for development of a sound working relationship between doctor and his or her patient "should take precedence over all other considerations" (APA 2001: 10, our emphasis).

In some other medical specialties, it must be granted, the *persona* of the practitioner may be just as important: primary care medicine is an obvious example. From the virtual absence of a doctor–patient relationship in pathology practice, to the transient, instrumentally driven relationships in radiological procedures, relations with patients are absent, time- or domain-limited, and relatively, although not absolutely, superficial, in many other medical specialties.

Traditionally, the dynamics of transference and counter-transference have been invoked to explain the force of remarks such as those in the *Annotations* (just as they have been to explain the increased power accorded to the practitioner in these settings [Phillips 1980–1981]). And indeed, in much theorizing about long-term psychodynamic psychotherapy, particularly, the resolution of the transference is regarded as necessary and even sufficient for healing. While many practitioners and patients would today challenge these assumptions and the theory from which such generalizations are derived, there remains widespread agreement, confirmed by empirical studies conducted during the 1970s and 1980s by the National Institute of Mental Health, that psychotherapeutic effectiveness depends, in some way, on the relationship or alliance between practitioner and patient. (See Elkin, Parloff, et al. 1985; Elkin, Pilkonis, et al. 1985; Elkin et al. 1989; Shea et al. 1992; Sotsky et al. 1991.) These studies were not primarily designed to establish this outcome; they were elaborately structured to compare forms of treatment that included psychopharmacology and cognitive therapy with solely interpersonal therapy (ITP). But the unexpectedly strong showing of ITP in comparison with those other forms of treatment nonetheless points to this conclusion. Moreover, though limited to patients suffering depression, the findings about the efficacy of the therapeutic relationship from these NIMH studies have been regarded as applicable to other disorder categories as well.

While its exact nature is not entirely understood, the part played by the practitioner's *persona* or self is usually taken to be a *sine qua non* of the therapeutic engagement (Dawes 1994; Frank and Frank 1991; Moerman 2002; Rogers 1957; Strupp 1986). (Clinical lore offers the motto: "You can only take a patient as far as you have gone" to illustrate this interconnection between the self of the practitioner and the possibility of therapeutic effectiveness.) In confirming the importance and efficacy of the therapeutic relationship, the NIMH studies used uniform, objective outcome measures. By contrast, earlier studies had explored the same issue from the perspective of patients' perception (Sloane et al. 1975). Those with successful outcomes rated the personal interaction with the therapist as the single most important factor in their treatment and, on a self-assessment of outcome, correlated success with the presence of higher levels of warmth, empathy, or genuineness in their therapists (Sloane et al. 1975: 225). The personal traits of the therapist were thus identified as the key ingredients marking therapeutic effectiveness. And even earlier, in an influential paper based on his clinical experience, Carl Rogers identified traits in the therapist that he believed were necessary and sufficient for therapeutically effected healing, or what he called "personality change": the genuineness and transparency he referred to as "congruence"; the attitudes of warmth, caring, liking, interest, and respect he entitled "unconditional positive regard," and finally, empathic understanding (Rogers 1957).

On this question not of whether, but of how, the therapeutic relationship heals, the most sustained and useful research is found in the work of Frank and Frank, introduced earlier. These authors have focused on identifying the ingredients in the effective therapeutic relationship. Study after study, they emphasize, has shown that "effectiveness is primarily a *quality of the therapist*, not of a particular technique" (Frank and Frank 1991: 166, our emphasis). They point to further ingredients of successful therapeutic outcomes, including structural aspects of the setting (such factors as a clearly defined healing space, and a ritual of some sort to bind the relationship between the healer and patient), and to aspects of the patient, including a readiness to be healed. But their primary emphasis is on personal qualities in the therapist, such traits as "persuasive talent and innate warmth" (Frank and Frank 1991: 100).

In rather similar work from the same era, four features of therapeutic effort have been hypothesized to explain successful therapeutic outcomes: guided by theory, therapists are motivated to persevere; they create and maintain an interpersonal context characterized by empathic listening; they seek to understand the meaning of the patient's inner states; and they attempt to reformulate these affectively charged meanings in a way that the patient can productively assimilate (Strupp 1986). Commenting on this research, Daniel Moerman has pointed out that to the extent that these four are the ingredients of therapeutic effectiveness, it must be in virtue of the meanings assigned to them by the patient (Moerman 2002: 95). This observation is surely correct, and as Moerman rightly emphasizes, it exposes the confused thinking around the assertion, sometimes voiced, that the effectiveness of the therapeutic alliance is a "mere" placebo effect.

This matter of the placebo effect is important, and deserves to be stressed. When compared with chemically active ingredients in a placebo-controlled study, placebo is chemically inert. But it is not always "inert" in the sense of without effectiveness—the placebo effect is so named, after all, because it is an effect. That effect, the result of the patient's understanding of what is experienced (or of "meanings," in Moerman's analysis) is the coin of the realm in any communicative, interpersonal relationship. The effect of psychotherapy is as real and powerful as—and no different from—any other change resultant from ordinary learning, that is, one person's understanding of his or her experience.

To the extent that the practitioner must utilize her own *persona* or self in the interests of achieving therapeutic effectiveness, this would seem to impose extra ethical responsibilities on the practitioner not required of those engaged in less personally involving forms of medical practice. Most generally, it will take extra attention to self-presentation, and to the impression and effects of one's words, gestures, demeanor, appearance, and behavior. Moreover, it will demand certain traits in the practitioner—traits such as warmth and empathy, if these studies are to be our guide. Certainly, we can see how some traits might be impediments to therapeutic effectiveness: the psychiatrist who has little tolerance for her own anxiety is unlikely to provide the necessary forbearance to an anxious patient; he who is unreflectively conventional will have difficulty accepting the idiosyncrasies of his patient suffering a schizotypal disorder.

Some might suppose the treatment model presupposed here is not as common as it once was; increasing reliance on psychopharmacology seems to be fast reducing access to in-depth, long-term, psychotherapy. Yet regardless of the truncated approach employed to bring about the goal, holistic and far-reaching conceptions of the patient and her life remain centrally embedded in that goal, we want to emphasize. And the project remains a normative one of profound social significance, as some more thoughtful proponents of the new approaches have demonstrated, especially in relation to the effects of the new psychopharmacologies. Peter Kramer early pointed out that fundamental questions of personal identity are raised by the capabilities of a new class of antidepressant medications and raise themselves in the therapeutic setting (Kramer 1993). And with Carl Elliott he has drawn attention to the broad, normative implications of drugs that, by blurring the boundary between healing and enhancement, complicate conceptions of health (Elliott and Kramer 2003).

Similarly, Nassir Ghaemi describes how for effective treatment, psychopharmacologists, too, must utilize their *persona* or self in treatment, marshalling feelings of empathy and their own existential despair. Empathy, Ghaemi notes, is an "essential psychotherapeutic aspect of psychiatric treatment;" for example, with patients, who suffer from "deadening world-views." It becomes the psychopharmacologist's task, he explains, by utilizing empathy, "to delve into [the patients'] worldviews, gain their trust, and slowly pull them out far enough so that they can see the need for treatment with medication. This task can be achieved by the use of our own existential despair...as a tool to contact patients ensconced in depressive world-views" (Ghaemi 2003: 285).

Rather than attached to a model that has outlived its usefulness, we believe that the features of the psychiatry setting described here still relate to the healing project, as well as to the nature of the therapeutic alliance. Indeed, they are intrinsic to it.

As was noted earlier, psychiatry is not the only medical specialty where a strong doctor–patient relationship is efficacious in healing and perhaps also, thus, ethically desirable. So this feature of the psychiatry setting may be judged one in which it is distinguished by degree rather than kind from other medical settings. That degree is nonetheless significant. Psychiatry is the only specialty where, in one of its therapeutic modes—psychotherapy—the use of the therapeutic alliance is regarded as not only necessary, but as alone sufficient, for healing.

Managed Care Delivery Systems

Managed care, at least in the United States, refers to private medical insurers' involvement with reimbursement for care, as well as the regulation of care delivery, quantity, and, often, quality. With its incumbent model of the patient as a consumer of medical services, managed care medicine may be expected, with time, to eradicate any lingering differences between psychiatry and other medicine. But we would challenge this assumption also. There is much suggesting that in the era of managed care delivery systems, psychiatry differs from the rest of medicine as much, or more, than before.

Recent critiques have made clear that managed care structures impose particular ethical strains on patient privacy and confidentiality of records (Alarcon 2000; Green 1999; Lazarus and Sharfstein 1998; Meyer and McLaughlin 1998; Morreim 1990; Schlesinger et al. 2000). Because of the social attitudes that continue to stigmatize mental disorder and psychiatric treatment, confidentiality takes on a unique ethical importance with the almost routinely sensitive and personal nature of the issues raised in treatment. The privacy violations likely to ensue will require extra vigilance and higher standards of confidentiality in this new context. Breaches of confidentiality have a direct bearing on treatment effectiveness in as much as they jeopardize the trust that the patient has in the practitioner, as these critiques have also illustrated. And because of the unparalleled importance of the therapeutic alliance in psychiatry, trust is an especially vital ingredient in that setting.

Because of their importance to much of the private practice of psychiatry in the United States today, we take up issues relating to managed care delivery systems throughout this book. (See Chapters 3, 5, and 6.) Our comments form a progressive argument, interwoven through the pages that follow, which fit in at different places for different reasons.

Managed care structures often impose multiple and potentially incompatible roles on practitioners: not only healer but cost cutter and social planner, for example, and steward of limited resources. And just as the dual roles imposed by society in asking the psychiatrist to protect the public as well as heal the patient, the multiple roles imposed by managed care have been recognized to increase the ethical dilemmas and quandaries for practitioners. In this respect, perhaps, managed care imposes ethical demands felt evenly across all medical specialties. These multiple roles and role quandaries must further jeopardize patient trust, however. And on account of the heightened need for trust in psychiatric practice (discussed more fully in Chapter 5) this becomes a pointed issue. Practitioners in psychiatry may thus be subject to greater demands in order to maintain the confidence and trust of their patients than will other practitioners in most, if not all, other medical specialties.

Managed care brings another, more general, ethical challenge as well. The same traits that render many psychiatric patients particularly vulnerable to exploitation are also those that, as we saw earlier, may limit the appropriateness of according to those patients full autonomy. These matters have profound implications in light of managed care, which is a system more wedded to the negotiated contract principle and the consumer model than previous systems of mental health care. Ethical managed care, we hope to demonstrate, must be sensitive to the possibility of differences between many psychiatric patients and other health care consumers, cognizant of the fluid and multifarious conflicts of duty and interest peculiar to mental health care, and respectful of the dangers of misapplying the consumer model to cases, and stages, of the patient's experience with mental disorder where they are inappropriate.

Community Psychiatry, Consumer Sensitivity, and the Survivor, Recovery, Users, and "Mad Pride" Movements

The user of mental health care provides a perspective absolutely invaluable to an understanding of psychiatric symptoms and mental health practice. This has implications for several practical and policy trends, including the inclusion on psychiatric ethics and human rights committees, policy-making bodies, and diagnostic manual committees of those who have experienced the system at first hand. Although the rhetoric from the various consumer movements diverges widely, not only in emphasis but in its substantive presuppositions and assertions, some broad claims of these several different groups and movements are shared. They urge that consumers be heard. They ask for an end to discrimination and prejudice. They ask to be recognized as autonomous persons and valued and respected as such. And they ask for a chance to participate in their recovery and in reshaping cultural ideas about mental health and illness.

The demands on the practitioner deriving from these shared ideas, and their ethical implications, seem fairly clear. To the extent that it is possible to listen for, hear, invite, and respect, the perspective of the patient, whether in the context of the therapeutic setting, or in these other settings where policy affecting the consumer is discussed, the clinician should make every effort to do so. Inasmuch as they will serve to prevent the voices of consumers from being heard, practice trends including the move away from lengthy interviews (often dictated by managed care economics), and the matching costs in interpersonal skills training in psychiatry education (growing from emphasis on the biomedical side of psychiatry), must be resisted.

The ideas and assumptions expressed by these welcome new movements deserve respect and serious consideration: consumers' voices must be heard. And the consumer slogan "Nothing about us without us,"[9] is one that should be honored. But the extent to which the ethical psychiatrist must adopt and accept each of the claims of those speaking from such a consumer perspective is not so apparent—in part because these several movements do not speak with one voice. Some rhetoric is vehemently "antipsychiatry," rejecting not only the label of sick patient, and the medical model underlying much contemporary psychiatric theorizing, but, as we noted earlier, the whole professional *raison d'être* of the practitioner. Other differences are less immediately incompatible with the practitioner's sense of profession and role. Yet they introduce quite fundamental—and sometimes entirely incompatible—assumptions about the nature of mental disorder. Consider, for example, presuppositions about psychiatric symptoms when the concern is to be acknowledged as a person distinct from, and not reducible to, the disorder (Deegan 2001). Definitions have been devised to accord with the sense of recovery as defining a self apart from symptoms (Barham 1997; Barham and Hayward 1991, 1995, 1998; Bracken and Thomas 2005; Corrigan and Penn 1998; Davidson 2003; Jacobson and Greenley 2001; Ridgeway 2001). In contrast, some in these movements present their symptoms as integral to their identity. They demand that we acknowledge their status as separate, and deeply different, yet deserving of equal respect and treatment. Some mad pride rhetoric analogizes madness with blackness, and links the efforts

[9] See Charlton (1998).

of activists to earlier civil rights movements. The disorder is even "valorized" and celebrated.[10]

The practitioner cannot be required to adopt such fundamentally warring sets of assumptions, not only because they are incompatible but because no one of them might correspond to her own views. But she can be asked to try to understand, and to respect, these alternative perspectives, recognizing the degree of controversy attaching to these ideas, and understanding the source of that controversy—the extent to which they rest not only on discoverable empirical realities but on deeply held moral and philosophical attitudes and beliefs. Accordingly, she can be expected to approach her own stance with an appropriate humility, allowing herself to meet the patient "where she is," and to negotiate treatment with explicit reference to the patient's values and perspective.

Conclusion

We have identified a number of intertwined aspects of the psychiatric setting each of which seems to contribute to separating psychiatry from other medical practices. These included aspects of the patient, symptoms and disorder; features of the societal structures within which psychiatry is today practiced, including managed care systems; facts about the historical and cultural origins of stigma and controversy, and of aspects of the healing project, including its holistic focus, and the part attributable to the therapeutic alliance. Each of these aspects of the psychiatric setting, we have shown, apparently generates its own additional ethical demands.

Taken alone, only one of these elements—the unfailing responsibility to seclude and treat patients without their consent—may be entirely distinct to psychiatric practice. (And even it, we saw, is dependent upon present mental

---

[10] Rather than regarding his schizophrenia symptoms as annoying traits to be managed and controlled, survivor Simon Morris celebrates them, remarking, "There is really so much that's positive and exciting about 'illnesses' like 'schizophrenia.' All of us who've experienced 'deep sea fishing' will know the sensation of heightened awareness, of consciousness enhanced far better than LSD could ever do it, of feelings of wonder and terror that can't be verbalized…I was always mad—I hope I always will be. My crazy life is wonderful. The 'sane' really don't know what they're missing" (Morris 2000: 207–208).

health policy, which might one day change.) The powerful uniqueness of psychiatry as social and medical practice derives from the combination of these elements. Their presence together in the psychiatry setting differentiates the practice of psychiatry enough from other branches of medicine for us to acknowledge its placing additional ethical demands on practice.

3 Psychiatric Ethics as Virtue Ethics

*The virtues arise in us neither by nature nor against nature, but
we are by nature able to acquire them, and reach our complete
perfection through habit.*

ARISTOTLE, *NICHOMACHEAN ETHICS*, BOOK 2: 1103A24.

Introduction

Thus far, our plea for a special ethics for psychiatry has been made without
much invoking, or depending on, the idea of virtues. We have pointed out
features of the psychiatry setting that combine to distinguish it from other
medical practice. And we illustrated how these seem to call for a special moral
focus and impose distinctive ethical challenges. The extra ethical demands,
conflicts, and dilemmas seen in the psychiatric setting could be approached
through the application of the four principles of autonomy, benevolence,
nonmaleficence, and justice, it is true, or, appealing to a traditional, Kantian
deontological ethical framework, by acknowledging extra ethical duties or
responsibilities they impose on the practitioner. (That said, we align ourselves
with many contemporary virtue theorists in believing that ultimately principles and duties can also been seen to derive from the character virtues of
individuals.) In this chapter the argument is taken another step: we show how
psychiatric ethics can—and should—be virtue based. Reasons are developed
to support our view that an emphasis on virtues would be particularly fitting
for the psychiatric setting.

We begin by introducing general features of virtue-based ethical
approaches. From these approaches, we will point to several facts that are

invited by the psychiatry setting: the emphasis on inner states and responses as well as outer behavior; the complete moral psychology that accommodates the full description of these inner states; acknowledgment of the affective components of virtues, especially called for by the practice setting, that do not submit to rules (they are "unruly," as we put it), although through time they can be effectively habituated along the lines Aristotle envisioned; and the flexibility and "partialist" rather than "impartialist" focus.

In writing about the professions, and medicine in particular, there is a long and rich tradition of construing good practice in virtue terms. So we also note some of these earlier discussions, which contain both reasons in support of applying the virtues to professional ethics most generally, and reasons showing why virtues have a particular place in medical care. Finally, three considerations are introduced, each based on features of the psychiatry setting noted in Chapters 1 and 2. The first of these is the centrality of the therapeutic relationship, which seems to call for a particular degree of personal warmth and emotional responsiveness in the character of the good psychiatrist; the second derives from the public role accorded to the psychiatrist, who, we argue, will need to go beyond duty in fostering, and conveying, the trait of propriety; and the third arises from the nature of today's bureaucratized care delivery systems, which call for several kinds of virtue in practitioners, including the supererogatory leadership qualities demanded to defend the fiduciary goals of medicine against the often competing goals of the organization.

Together, these considerations seem to us to provide good reason to adopt a virtue ethics approach.

Virtue-Based Ethical Approaches

The framework or approach known as virtue ethics is usually placed in contrast to Kantian and Utilitarian systems. An *aretaic* or virtue-based ethics is one in which it is the self or character of the person that is the central focus of moral assessment, rather than particular actions or their consequences. Personal qualities such as honesty, integrity, courage, fairness, and compassion are to be found in the dispositions and responses of persons possessing good characters. Such character traits are the basis from which rights and duties are derived. Rights and duties are in this sense "derivative."

In Western traditions, virtue-based approaches to the moral life origi-nate with Greek philosophy and are particularly associated with Aristotle's *Nichomachean Ethics*; they are also found in medieval and eighteenth-century writing—including that of David Hume, which we will discuss later in this book. And they have seen a remarkable resurgence in the last decades of the twentieth century.[1] (See, for example, Compte-Spoonville 2001; Crisp 1996; Crisp and Slote 1997; Foot 1978; Hursthouse 1999; McDowell 1979; Oakley 1996; Pence 1991; Pincoffs 1986; Slote 2004; Stohr and Wellman 2002; Watson 1990; Williams 1986.) As this legacy suggests, virtue ethics is less one particular account of the moral life and moral value than a cluster of accounts, loosely united by their approach, but varying considerably in their details.

Virtues are stable dispositions or character traits. Once acquired, they are like good habits. And the process of cultivating virtues, like that of culti-vating any habits, is (at least as we understand it from Aristotle) incremental and un-heroic. It calls for attention, repetition, conscientiousness, and prac-tice. It is because of this emphasis on habituation in virtue ethics that we shall stress the applicability of this ethical framework for the educational setting in which practitioners are undergoing training in their specialty. The demands of virtue ethics very often function less as rules and more as ideals to be striven for and idealized character models to be emulated (see Pence 1991; Watson 1990).[2]

The contrast between prescriptions over particular actions, and pre-scriptions about more holistic and enduring traits, has been represented as something like: "*Do* thus and so," rather than the virtue-focused "*Be* thus and so." This emphasis on *being* a virtuous person by possessing a particu-lar character, rather than *doing* right action, does not imply that action or results secured by action are insignificant. Nonetheless, this is quite a deep difference. For instance, possessing a virtue might affect not how one acts

---

[1] Although they are not our focus here, non-Western traditions such as Confucianism also employ virtue-based ethical systems. (See Ivanhoe and Van Norden 2001; Yearley 1990.)

[2] Exploring the contrast between rules and ideals, Rosemary Tong remarks: "Whereas rules tell us what is forbidden, permitted, or required, and threaten us with sanc-tions for noncompliance, ideals encourage us…This is not to suggest that, com-pared to laws, ideals are a weak means of 'behavior control'. If an ideal takes over one's life, it can effect changes that no set of rules, however clearly enunciated and strictly enforced, can ever hope to effect" (Tong 1988: 89). That said, some virtue ethics has also been understood in terms of rules.

so much as how one responds emotionally in a particular situation. (Does a person feel indignation on witnessing injustice, for example, or remain indifferent?) It might express itself in a particular frame of mind or style of deliberation. (Some people measure, wait and withhold judgment; others jump to conclusions. Some need to see, others can imagine.) Or it might be identified not with a particular action so much as with a particular motive. (Even when outwardly identical, acts stemming from compassion and self-interest, respectively, differ in this way.) Speaking of the virtues in Greek philosophy, Terence Irwin has explained that virtue is not identified solely as something that makes you act the right way. We care about the virtuous character, he notes, "for its own sake apart from the behavioral result...We care about what people—ourselves and others—are like, and not simply what they do" (Irwin 1996: 47).

This more inward aspect of virtues seems to us central to the main argument of this book—that ethical psychiatry involves the character of the psychiatrist. In addition to the knowledge and skill demanded by the psychiatrist's role are feelings, and emotional attitudes, and responses that are conveyed not only through words but also through such nonverbal attributes as demeanor and body language—empathic listening, for example. Inner states, and dispositions to feel and respond in particular ways, and the ability to convey these nonverbally, are essential to fostering and maintaining the alliance that we have seen is necessary for effective practice.

As composites or trait clusters, virtues often comprise affective as well as more cognitive and motivational elements, of course, and these affective elements will not be as subject to immediate control as are many other responses. From virtue to virtue, the balance of ingredients, between more and less cognitive or affective, and controllable or uncontrollable, varies. Notably though, several of the key qualities called for by the psychiatry setting are primarily affective, making it difficult to accommodate them in rule-based ethical systems. They elude immediate control and are, or are partially, "unruly," in the sense that the responses they require cannot be invoked directly. Empathy is an example of such a trait—we cannot command ourselves to feel empathy. Similarly "unruly," and another attribute of the greatest importance to the therapeutic relationship, is genuine and spontaneous warmth. (This quality is discussed at more length later in the present chapter.) The unruly nature of several qualities of character required for effective treatment in the psychiatry setting is a central reason why we favor a virtue-based approach to psychiatric ethics.

Aristotle's account recognizes the importance of feelings as ingredients, and antecedents, of other moral virtues. But in our insistence that affective states such as empathy and warmth are themselves virtues, we are closer to the eighteenth-century philosopher Hume, for whom primarily affective states such as benevolence and compassion were not only important virtues in their own right but, indeed, central to all moral response. Hume believed, and much recent research seems to confirm, that these affections are based on a natural tendency to recognize others' inner states and respond sympathetically. (We return to this matter in discussion of empathy and compassion in Chapter 5.) Unlike more traditional virtues, unruly states cannot be directly, voluntarily invoked, for all that they may stem from these natural tendencies, however. And to be realized, as Aristotle saw, they will need the appropriate reinforcement and education in childhood and youth. Still, adults are able to deepen and enhance the dispositions making up such virtues as empathy (Larson and Yao 2005). The tendency to respond with increased empathy can be engendered *indirectly*—by practicing certain habits of mind such as imaginatively placing ourselves in the situation of the other, and engaging in allied forms of simulation, and by paying close attention to the details of the other's hardship or plight. (We return to these habits of mind that comprise and engender feelings of empathy in Chapter 5.)

Reviewing types of virtue ethics, Justin Oakley has listed some additional features common to the traditions we are introducing here (Oakley 1996).[3] One is that goodness is said to be prior to rightness. This means the rightness of actions is to be identified through, and cannot be determined until we know, what is valuable or good. Another is that the virtues are irreducibly plural, intrinsic goods. This is in contrast to the reductive, instrumental view of goods held by Utilitarianism. In virtue theory, separate virtues are valued, each its own way, and not because of any relation it might bear to other goods such as happiness. Finally, some intrinsic goods are said to be agent-relative. A right response might be a reflection of the particular and idiosyncratic character of each individual and her relationships, and not be applicable to others' situations. (We return to this kind of partialism later in this chapter.)

On an Aristotelian schema there are several kinds of virtues, not all of which are the moral virtues of character. Some are intellectual virtues; others

---

[3] Oakley's full list includes six characteristics, but we have noted only those relevant to our immediate purposes.

are prudential virtues—useful for furthering one's interests. In this book we diverge from some of the details of Aristotle's account. For instance, traits, which for Aristotle, are not moral virtues (or in some cases not virtues of any kind), *become moral virtues when they are exercised as part of a professional role.* Thus, the particular virtues explored in the *Nichomachean Ethics*, such as temperance, generosity, courage, friendliness, justice, and continence, are not privileged in our discussion.[4] Certainly some of these traditional virtues are important to psychiatric practice; moreover, we shall pay particular attention to the Aristotelian virtue of *phronesis* (translated as practical wisdom or intelligence) because of its special applicability to practical action. But our discussion will also introduce valuable attributes not traditionally recognized as virtues, maintaining that, within the practice setting, those attributes acquire the status of role-constituted virtues.

More generally, we would emphasize, because virtue ethics involves everyday conduct, behaving virtuously means everyday conduct is laden with morality. Rather than requiring prescriptions that are esoteric or new, behaving virtuously means that everyday clinical practices and strategies can be understood as imbued with virtues.

The notion of character, so central to virtue ethics, is a complex and ambiguous one, and requires some clarification before we proceed further. Character sometimes refers to the set of a person's moral virtues (as in "She was a woman of character"); sometimes to his or her vices as well (as in "What bad characters they proved to be"). Even more broadly understood, character is sometimes equated with personality, and depicted as comprising a range of characteristic traits—positive, negative, and morally neutral. Thus, for example, Joel Kupperman treats the evaluative component as a matter of emphasis only, defining character as a normal pattern of thought and action (for any given person X who possesses that character) "*especially* with respect to concerns and commitments in matters affecting the happiness of others or of X, and *most especially* in relation to moral choices" (Kupperman 1991: 17, our emphasis). The same ambiguity is encountered, and perpetuated, in Christopher Peterson and Martin Seligman's recent study of character strengths (Peterson and Seligman 2004). Character strengths are defined as the psychological ingredients—processes or mechanisms—that define the virtues; virtues are said to be the core characteristics valued by

---

[4] As philosophers have shown, the virtues Aristotle selects for discussion are disappointingly elitist and sexist in some of their assumptions (Exdell 1987; Okin 1989, 1996).

moral philosophers and religious thinkers (Peterson and Seligman 2004: 13). Interestingly, on a common contemporary interpretation even Aristotle's *arête*, once regularly translated as "virtue," is rendered with the broader "excellence" to indicate that it spans both moral virtues and additional non-moral traits (Irwin 1985; Kupperman 1991).[5]

Whether or not we allow character to comprise evaluatively neutral traits as well as moral virtues (and or vices), and whatever way we understand the Aristotelian term *arête*, this set of distinctions proves insufficient when we turn to the traits that are part of the role morality of the ethical practitioner. Such role morality requires us to understand the designations "moral virtue" and "morally neutral trait" to be relational, so that *within the professional context*, any trait may *acquire the status* of a moral virtue.

In most traditional accounts of virtues each virtue is opposed to, and is a remedy against, a particular vice.[6] One's possession of the virtue of courage will help prevent one from succumbing to cowardice, the virtue of kindness to cruelty, the virtue of temperance to lust, and so on. On this model, virtues are "solutions to design flaws in human beings," as Julia Driver puts it (Driver 1996: 112): were there not particular human appetites, temptations, and weaknesses, they would be unnecessary.[7]

Following this model, there will be situation-specific vices or temptations, to which the role-constituted virtues identified here correspond, and against which they should serve as antidotes. Some of these temptations associated with the psychiatrist's role were introduced earlier, and we believe this an important and valuable aspect of virtue-based accounts in application to psychiatric ethics. (See Chapter 1.) Noting the opportunities for unethical behavior in the psychiatry setting, we pointed out that unethical responses are invited by features such as the vulnerabilities of patients, and the privacy of the arrangements governing therapeutic sessions, so that they apparently call for additional virtue, or an especially strong moral character, in practitioners. We return to these temptations when, in Chapter 5, we consider some of the role-constituted virtues called for by the psychiatric setting. This emphasis on the whole psychology of the moral life, and not merely

---

[5] This translation has been challenged (Beresford 2005).

[6] This is part of the Stoic-Christian-Kantian tradition only, according to Harris, and less true of Hellenistic conceptions (Harris 1979).

[7] It should be added that Driver is critical of this model, believing it mistaken in its presuppositions about human psychology and indeed in the presumption that a virtue theory could be grounded on any human psychology. (See Driver 1996: Chapter 3.)

on actions or their consequences, is a further reason that the language and structure of virtue ethics accommodates the introspective and inward nature of the practitioner—and project—in psychiatry.

Aristotle's virtues are linked to his teleological conception of human flourishing more generally understood. Some modern day virtue theorists accept this link also, believing that while it is not the *reason* we should be virtuous, the best outcomes, and a life most satisfactorily realized, will result from the cultivation of a virtuous character (McDowell 1979; Megone 2000).[8] Although some philosophers have seen a special applicability to modern day psychiatric practice in this aspect of Aristotelian theory, it will not be dealt with fully in what follows.

The central argument of this book is that a collection of features, jointly distinguishing the psychiatric setting, invites an ethics distinctive to psychiatry, and that a virtue-based framework well fits that need. More principle and rule-focused approaches such as Utilitarianism, or Kantianism, we believe, can be seen as derived from an analysis in terms of virtues. It is evident, for instance, that principle-based ethical systems of the kind introduced in Chapter 1, can readily be cast in virtue terms: the practitioner who values beneficence, for example, is one who possesses the virtue of beneficence; respect for autonomy is found in the possession of the virtue of respectfulness of others' autonomy, and so on. Interpretations of both Utilitarianism and Kantianism have also worked to accommodate an emphasis on character, arguing, respectively, that the nature and structure of a person's dispositions and character must be such as to maximize utility (Crisp 1992; Foot 1978; Railton 1988), and that something like Kant's categorical imperative is a normative disposition in the character of a good agent to rule out certain courses of action as impermissible (Herman 1993). Similarly, some versions of an ethics of care have been shown able to accommodate a focus on the character of the carer (Slote 2004). And even a pragmatist approach to ethical practice such as has recently been put forward by David Brendel, can be depicted in terms of the character traits of flexibility, sensitivity to context, and open-mindedness we associate with the pragmatist frame of mind (Brendel 2006).

[8] For a recent discussion of the central weakness of the virtues/flourishing link, see Stohr and Wellman (2002). As these authors remark, "unless a virtue ethicist can explain why, contrary to appearances, it is in an individual's interest to be just, there will remain a difference between the list of character traits required for moral behavior and those conducive to a good life" (Stohr and Wellman 2002: 66). (See also Hursthouse 1999.)

We are persuaded by the noteworthy fit between virtue-based systems and some of particular demands of the psychiatry setting, and we believe that ultimately, rules and principles derive from virtues. But we do not intend to exclude the use of rules and principles that might be necessary in accommodating the complex and multifaceted challenges set by the practice of psychiatry. An approach to identifying actions as either required, forbidden, or permitted, remains essential in codifying the minimally acceptable conduct in the relationship between the psychiatrist and patient, for example, if only for purposes of professional censure. Such language will also help establish minimal standards of professional practice. And, at the practical level, a focus on virtues will likely find its greatest usefulness in psychiatric education, and as an expression of the broad *ethos* of practice.

Virtues, Professionalism, and the Good Doctor

The concept of a virtuous character has been portrayed as central to professionalism (Dyer 1999; Kronman 1987; Moore and Sparrow 1990; Oakley and Cocking 2001). Traits such as trustworthiness, fidelity, honesty, and integrity have even been identified with professional status. To have a profession, as distinct from having mere technique, it has been said, implies "the possession of certain character-defining traits or qualities" (Kronman 1987: 841). The most helpful recent explication of this point of view is that of Justin Oakley and Dean Cocking, who offer a thoroughgoing account of why virtue ethics allows us to understand the nature and moral significance of professional roles (Oakley and Cocking 2001).

This position presupposes role morality. Professionals' roles call for extra virtue or extra virtues in their characters, distinguishing them, in the virtues demanded, from nonprofessional roles. (Notice that these demands do not require professionals to do, or to be, anything that conflicts with broad-based morality, as the more controversial strong role morality might do.)

This argument for the applicability of virtue and character ethics to professional practices may perhaps extend beyond medicine and law, but it is limited to "good professions"—those committed to a key human good which, as Oakley and Cocking say, plays a crucial role in "enabling us to live a humanly flourishing life" (Oakley and Cocking 2001: 74). Medicine unquestionably meets this standard. And qualities of character, as well as skill and learning, have always been acknowledged to be part of being a good doctor. As James Drane puts it, from the time of Hippocrates "medical codes have appealed for both *rules and virtue*" (our emphasis). Patients were expected to trust their physicians and to follow their advice because "doctors were persons of *excellent character.*" Indeed, superior moral development was considered to be "more important than following rules and regulations" (Drane 1995: 6–7).

Why should medical practices particularly invite an emphasis on virtues in their practitioners? One answer is put forward by Drane. The doctor is bound to higher ideals and higher virtues than other people, he remarks, because of the nature of the medical relationship. The clinical setting, for example, offers "existential situations." It calls for responses "along the line of cultivated attitudes and habits; that is, virtue and character responses," rather than permitting "objective facts [and]...objective rules for the right thing to do" (Drane 1995: 18). Such rules, he implies, would be blunt, inflexible, and inhumane for dealing with the complex and emotionally nuanced relationship between doctor and patient and the frequently serious nature of the patient's concerns. (Notice that Drane speaks of the cultivation of *attitudes* and habits. As we saw earlier, the dispositions making up virtues include several affective responses, emotions, feelings, and attitudes. Drane recognizes that such affective states are an integral part of many important doctors' virtues.)

One of the major reasons virtue ethics has been seen as an appealing alternative to Kantianism and Utilitarianism is that the kind of "impartialism" integral to, and lauded in, both these other frameworks has come to be regarded as an impoverished and even wrongful picture of the moral life and moral deliberation (Williams 1986). Some of our central human roles and activities seem to require not an impartial but a partial response toward others. It is recognized, for example, that a parent will, and *should*, prefer his or her own children's welfare and safety to that of other children. And we can see that the same seems true in the relationship between practitioner and patient: the practitioner's preference for the interests and well-being of his or her own particular patients is a mainstay of the professional role. This critique emphasizes the irreducibly particular nature of the ethical choices and situations that arise in health care. We sometimes cannot and, more important, we should not, act impartially as traditional Kantian and Utilitarian ethical systems seem to require. "[R]ole specific duties are incurred precisely out of one's status and function as a physician," as Churchill has put it, and those duties pertain to "my patients, persons who occupy a special, especially vulnerable position and with whom I have enacted special ties and bonds" (Churchill 1989: 28–29).

The practitioner–patient relationship at the heart of any type of medical practice demands partial, not impartial, responses from the practitioner then, and a virtue ethical framework, it has been supposed, best accommodates this partial approach. Whether this is a reason to see virtue ethics as having particular application to mental health care, rather than health care more generally, is arguable.[9] But whatever its other applications, virtue ethics' accommodation of partial, rather than impartial, responses from the practitioner is indeed a strong reason to apply virtue ethics to the psychiatry setting.

Some Misgivings about Virtue Talk

A tendency toward platitudes seems to be a special risk with talk of virtues. Unlike other ethical systems and approaches, virtue ethics can seem so vague and general as to be close to vacuous. Action guiding rules about what is permitted, required, and forbidden, for example, or reference to a single principle such as that of utility, give us something clear and specific to bring to cases and dilemmas. By contrast, appeals to virtues seem abstract and elusive. Virtue concepts, like compassion, beneficence, or justice, appear to be abstractions, also. The dispositions such concepts embody may be interpreted and manifest in any number of ways (consider, for example, the multitude of ways the disposition to benevolence might be made manifest); in their generality they overlap and blur together, so that the substantive difference between say, trustworthiness, fidelity, and moral integrity, would be difficult to specify. Virtue language is confusingly ambiguous, in addition: to attribute virtue is sometimes to imply exceptional virtue, yet there is an expectation that the usual virtues will be exhibited, from time to time, by everyone (Blum 2007: 235). Some of this vagueness and ambiguity derives from the way virtues function as goals to strive for, rather than concrete rules. Virtue, as Dyer puts it, aspires to ideals, which cannot be perfectly met, in contrast to the "accountability" that holds someone to a standard that has been explicitly specified. Virtue is "lofty, even precarious" (Dyer 1999: 74).

Virtue ethics may seem somewhat unsatisfactory in another way. In traditional virtue theory, we know a person is benevolent, for example, because he acts in a kindly way. Our attribution to that person of benevolence is *reliant* on the way it is manifested in observable behavior. His benevolence has

[9] This view has been expressed by Crowden (2003).

objective status, according to virtue theorists. And because virtues are called for only by specific, appropriate occasions, which may not actually arise, it will be possible to possess benevolence without manifesting it on any particular occasion. So when we attribute virtues, we do so from a state of some epistemic disadvantage. Like the signs and symptoms of disease, the outer evidence of virtue does not provide an entirely dependable basis for attributing the moral trait.

Combined with these epistemic vagaries, the vagueness noted above makes it easy to dismiss as perhaps true, but entirely *unhelpful,* the claim that practitioners must possess particular virtues or be especially virtuous. And some previous writing in which ethical behavior for professionals has been understood within a virtue framework has tended toward such vagueness and vacuity.[10]

Our goal here is to go beyond platitudes about virtue and in so doing demonstrate a virtue ethics framework to full advantage by showing the reasons why the particular practice of psychiatry requires particular attributes in its practitioners. To do this, it is necessary to examine the responses called for by the practice setting (the setting that includes the disorder, the social and cultural context, the healing project, and so on), and to show how each response can be linked to particular virtues in the character of the ethical practitioner. Another way to say this is that *the setting provides moral reasons for the practitioner to be, and to respond, in certain ways.* By linking the aspects of the practice setting with the character of the psychiatrist and so showing why and how the practitioner must possess both uncommon virtues and uncommon virtue, we hope to move beyond platitudes and provide a substantive and useful portrait of the virtuous psychiatrist.[11]

[10] In a related problem there appears to be no independent way to specify what virtue is other than by appeal to the nature of virtuous people. (See Hursthouse 1999.)

[11] In a critique of virtue ethics, Veatch has placed in contrast human contacts between strangers and those between intimates and members of communities "sharing a common vision." In health care practice, which is among strangers, he insists, there can be no shared understanding of the virtuous life, thus virtues must at best be understood as having instrumental value (Veatch 1988: 466). Even in some less personal medical practices (where "strangers" may be applicable), it is arguable that some shared vision of health and well-being unites doctor and patient. But in the practice of psychiatry, this is an inapplicable model on every count. Aspects of the project of psychiatry, including the way it is effected through personal relationship, it involves feelings and disclosures of the most personal and private kind,

The Virtuous Psychiatrist

Inasmuch as they deal with the virtues of all professionals, analyses such as Oakley and Cocking's have valuable application to psychiatry. In contrast to the rich tradition of writing about the virtuous doctor, however, the particular character of the virtuous psychiatrist has received rather scant attention. Exceptions include sustained work by Dyer, to which we have referred already, by Andrew Crowden, and by Beauchamp (Beauchamp 1999; Crowden 2003; Dyer 1999; Mann 1997).

Beauchamp's remarks about why a virtuous character in the practitioner may be requisite for ethical psychiatric practice underscore our earlier emphasis on the affective nature of some virtues. Whenever the feelings, concerns, and attitudes of others are the morally relevant matters (as they are, Beauchamp implies, in psychiatry), then as he puts it "rules and principles are not as likely as human warmth and sensitivity to lead a person to notice what should be done." From this perspective, virtue ethics is "at least as fundamental in the moral life as principles of basic obligation" (Beauchamp 1999: 30).

This passage reminds us of an aspect of the psychiatry setting noted earlier, where we saw that personal warmth in the practitioner was cited as key to therapeutic effectiveness. (See Chapter 2.) In psychiatry, Beauchamp implies, the feelings, concerns, and attitudes of others are morally relevant matters and this is more true, or true more often, than in other professional, or even many other medical, settings. Only by possessing the traits of warmth and sensitivity could a person be led to take the right action in such delicate, emotionally charged, and significant human encounters as regularly occur in the psychiatric setting. If warmth and sensitivity are rightly described as virtues—and, we insist, they are—then the virtuous psychiatrist who possessed them would likely be a more effective practitioner than the virtue-less one who did not.

Beauchamp offers a brief sketch of a kind of empty obedience that would reveal, in his words, a person who was "morally lacking": he describes those who "always perform obligations because they are obligations, but who ... do not cherish, feel congenial toward, or think fondly of others, and treat them as they should only because obligation requires it." As psychiatrists, such

it is potentially long-term treatment due to the nature of severe mental disorder, and it addresses and interrogates the patient's values and visions of the good life, all combine to make it close to relationships with those sharing a common vision encompassing every aspect of life and experience.

persons would likely be without the "admirable compassion, commitment, and conscientiousness" guiding the lives of many dedicated health professionals (Beauchamp 1999: 30). This portrait of the virtue-less practitioner may be something of a caricature. Yet the passage is telling because of Beauchamp's emphasis on the quality of warmth that is believed to be so important in the therapeutic encounter. Beauchamp seems to recognize that, unlike some of the other responses he notes, including sensitivity, warmth is an unruly attitude. The genuine warmth found in the dedicated professional Beauchamp describes comes from deep within her character. It results not from following rules but from traits so internalized that (in certain situations) they give rise to spontaneous responses. Unruly responses such as these, we saw, cannot become an ingrained part of one's character through any direct exercise of will. We cannot admonish ourselves to respond warmly any more than we can to feel empathy. The best we can ask ourselves is to appear to respond warmly. Affected, studied, or feigned warmth is unlikely to be as effective as unfeigned warmth in the therapeutic context, however. (We return to the issue of feigned responses and feigned virtues in Chapter 6.) The warmth required here is genuine warmth. And indeed, as we saw earlier, several analyses of the *persona* of the practitioner identify genuineness as one of the handful of traits essential to effective healing (Frank and Frank 1991; Rogers 1957; Sloane et al. 1975). Apparently pointing to the same quality of genuineness, naturalness, or spontaneity, Carl Rogers described a trait involving "congruence" between inner feelings and outer displays; Frank and Frank speak of the need for responses that are "innate."

In some circumstances, at least, and in normal personal relationships, most people will surely be capable of feeling and conveying some degree of personal warmth. But for the enhanced degree of warmth required by the practice setting in psychiatry, repetition and practice will likely be needed. This, we saw, is also true of empathy. And, indeed, it is unclear whether we are considering two distinct sets of responses when speaking of personal warmth and empathy, or one that is variously construed and characterized. In his work on the importance to moral performance of emotions that allow us to encounter others as emotional beings, Arne Vetlesen uses the collective expression "empathic emotions," and, because of the similarities between the responses we have thus far distinguished as empathy and personal warmth, respectively, this general term covers both responses (Vetlesen 1994). Like that of habituating other such empathic emotions (to borrow Vetlesen's term), the task of habituating this augmented degree of personal warmth must be undertaken indirectly through the exercise of capabilities like attention and the imagination that are subject to will. Such indirect alteration of one's feelings, attitudes, and inner responses can involve redescribing the other person, for example, as well as variously simulating that person's own states (Blum 1980; Gordon 1995; Ickes 1997; Murdoch 1967).

It should be added here that between unruly virtues such as empathy and personal warmth lie at least some intermediate traits, which are more open to habituation on the standard model. Hopefulness is an example of one of these. We cannot instruct ourselves to be hopeful: "Be hopeful" no—but "*Try* to be hopeful" yes, and "Look on the bright side" yes. Certain *habits* of mind seem to be recognized to engender the right *frame* of mind, suggesting that these are habits that work, and frames of mind that we, too, can adopt through habituation.

Two further aspects of these particular unruly virtues need clarification: their expression in demeanor and body language, and the incremental nature of their habituation.

Although affective states are usually depicted as inner states, and not mere dispositions to act, it nonetheless remains true that traits such as spontaneous warmth are not merely inner states. They have important *outward* manifestations. They show themselves not only in actions but in demeanor and body language, for example. It will be insufficient, then, that the practitioner possesses the requisite degree of genuine feelings of warmth toward her patient; this must be made evident to the patient. Moreover, the demand that personal warmth be "genuine," "natural," "innate," or "spontaneous" adds something else. Their characteristic unruliness again appears in the way emotional states manifest themselves, which differs from the more studied communicative responses associated with speech and action. The public and observable manifestations of emotional responses are said to be "evinced" or "expressed" with the suggestion that, just as we cannot completely command our affective life, we cannot entirely control their expression.

Most forms of emotional expression are culturally shaped, it can be granted. Nonetheless, long habituation produces an involuntary quality that is captured in this demand for "natural" or "spontaneous" expression: if not quite natural, such expression can become "second nature." Apart from the indirect way they must be habituated required by their nature as unruly virtues, it must now be emphasized, achieving the personal warmth and empathy we have deemed key role specific virtues here will likely take time, perhaps even more than is required for the habituation of other virtues.

Although virtuous, the person who has intentionally manipulated feelings to make himself or herself respond warmly may not yet fully possess the appealing quality of naturalness we associated with genuine warmth. Only long cultivated habits such as these will bring about the enhanced degree of spontaneous warmth that is part of the character of the ethical psychiatrist and finds this kind of "natural" expression in her demeanor. As this indicates, genuine warmth is better understood as an ideal to be striven after, than a duty, or a milestone to be achieved. The seasoned virtuous practitioner will exceed the novice in the depth and genuineness of this trait.

Reprising this discussion of Beauchamp's example of genuine warmth, we want to stress that the psychiatry setting (in particular the demands upon the practitioner in developing and fostering the therapeutic alliance or relationship) calls for a heightened degree of such unruly attitudes and emotional responses. These responses bespeak underlying dispositions to respond, or qualities of character, rather than obedience to rules. We regard this as one of several important reasons why a virtue-based approach is particularly fitting for the psychiatry setting.

Role Constituted Virtues

Whatever traits and dispositions are called for by the psychiatry setting *or instrumental in promoting healing* become what we call in this book role-constituted virtues. In everyday contexts, personal warmth, for example, is a trait not universally supposed a moral virtue. (Arguably, it ought to be. But that is not a position we will adopt here. In our society, at least, personal warmth is unevenly admired, and its value is context and social role specific.) Yet, as we saw above, it appears to be such a role-constituted virtue. To better see how this is so, it will be helpful to return to role morality and to develop more fully our new theoretical construct of role-constituted virtues and their corresponding, setting-specific vices or temptations.

To ensure conduct and dispositions conducive to the particular good of that profession, each profession will honor and maintain certain standards. Professional ideals are "regulative," as Oakley and Cocking put it. Most generally understood, the promotion of health is the good, and regulative ideal, of healing practices; for the practitioner in psychiatry, this becomes the promotion of mental or psychological health. Understood within a virtue ethics framework, this good is sought through the cultivation of those traits and disposition that promote healing and mental health. And if certain dispositions and responses are required for, and or markedly enhance, the effectiveness of treatment in psychiatry, the ethical psychiatrist will need to possess those dispositions and responses in order to maximize therapeutic effectiveness. While not all are virtues outside of the professional context (and certainly not all are Aristotelian moral virtues, for instance), these traits are part of the professional's moral character, and the imperative to cultivate and exercise them is a moral one. As Oakley and Cocking put it: "on a virtue ethics approach to professional roles, something can be a virtue in professional life—such as a doctor's acute clinical judgment in making a correct diagnosis from a multitude of symptoms—*which might be neutral in ordinary life*" (Oakley and Cocking 2001: 129, our emphasis).

Peterson and Seligman separate virtues from the capabilities or "character strengths" into which they may be analyzed (Peterson and Seligman 2004). But, to return to the example of personal warmth, even if in everyday settings warmth were taken to be a virtue of some nonmoral kind (perhaps a prudential virtue), it nonetheless is made up of traits that are unequivocally neutral in ordinary life. Imaginative flexibility, a comfort with expressing and conveying feelings, a ready empathy, an ability to identify emotional saliencies in others, probably a skill at reading others' extra-verbal expressions, a quickness to respond emotionally, skills at the language of gesture, and so on, are not generally deemed valuable in themselves, only useful in certain settings and roles. Yet to the extent that they comprise what we recognize as personal warmth, these traits are, or are part of, role-constituted virtues.

A partial definition by virtue theorist Alasdair MacIntyre asserts that virtue is "an acquired human quality the possession and exercise of which tends to enable us to achieve those goods which are internal to practices and the lack of which effectively prevents us from achieving any such goods" (MacIntyre 1984: 178). As a definition of virtues in all spheres of life, this will be insufficient, and it has been criticized because of its narrowly instrumentalist emphasis (Crisp and Slote 1997: 11–13; Pincoffs 1986: 96). Yet this instrumentalist emphasis is precisely what fits this account as a definition for the role-constituted virtues of interest to us. Warmth and its cluster of subtraits, like the traits comprising sensitivity, are role constituted virtues in being *qualities the possession and exercise of which tend to enable us to achieve those goods that are internal to professional practice.*

The affective nature, and consequent unruliness, of some of the traits called for in the therapeutic relationship constitute one important reason why a virtue-based approach is particularly fitting for the psychiatry setting: several of its role-constituted virtues are traits requiring long and indirect habituation. Further reasons are outlined in the rest of this chapter, corresponding to two features of the psychiatry setting introduced in Chapter 2. The first is the special societal role imposed on the practitioner with the power of civil commitment that, we argue, demands the attention to appearances here named the virtue of propriety. The second concerns some self-unifying and leadership virtues apparently called for by today's managed care delivery systems.

Supererogatory Demands: Publicly Appearing As Well As Being Virtuous

Of the several aspects combining to distinguish psychiatry from other kinds of medical practice, one is the special power accorded to the psychiatrist by society in secluding and treating adults against their wishes for others', and their own, protection. The role of other medical practitioners in this duty varies, but the licensed psychiatrist is in many settings the sole medical practitioner responsible for such commitment.

The moral and political significance of this exception is enormous. In a constitutional democracy such as ours with a massive bulwark protecting innocent adults' individual liberty, this is a quite remarkable degree of power. It has few analogies. (Police powers, equally extensive, are the obvious ones.) Following some suggestion in the writing of Fraser, we earlier sketched the view that this extraordinary societal role imposes extra ethical demands on the psychiatrist exceeding those applicable to other medical practitioners.

As well as calling for virtue, these unique powers call for something like the appearance of virtue or at the least an avoidance of the appearance of vice, as we noted earlier. Entrusted with the power of civil commitment the psychiatrist must meet the ethical demands of the immediate situation but at the same time convey to the public that such virtue is being upheld.

That their societal role may require certain professionals not only to conduct themselves ethically but to avoid exhibiting or conveying the appearance of misconduct is an idea familiar from the "appearance" and conflict of interest standards sometimes imposed on those in government office. Because of the mere appearance of impropriety it conveys, public officials are prevented from accepting large contributions from interested individuals. Applied to elected officials, the appearance standard has been provided with several rationales. The most distinctive of these involves the maintenance of public confidence and trust. The legislator who accepts a large contribution from a constituent with an obvious interest is guilty of failing to take into account his constituency's reasonable reactions. This high standard is required, it is said, because citizens are not in a position to find out when and whether elected representatives take advantage of their position to act unethically.[12]

Although their temptations may be different, the government official's role bears significant parallels that of the psychiatrist participating in involuntary confinement and treatment. Like all government servants, the psychiatrist acts as society's representative in this role. Citizens have an interest in the confinement of the dangerous mentally ill and benefit from the public safety that is the goal of such confinement. For public safety and peace of mind, they must have complete confidence in the judgment and trustworthiness of the professionals who accept on their behalf this serious, but necessary, duty. Ordinary citizens are also unable to find out or judge for themselves whether any given civil commitment decision arbitrarily exceeds the exercise of power it involves. (This is additionally true in the psychiatric case, where professional expertise and technical skill guide such decisions.) Thus, they must trust psychiatric practitioners. Maintaining that trust in practitioners is essential for the maintenance of these necessary societal structures.

Arguably, then, it will behoove practitioners in psychiatry to avoid the public appearance of unethical conduct. As societal representatives authorized to override the civil liberty of a person not guilty or even suspected of crimes, psychiatrists must not only do the right thing, but also uphold the public trust imposed on them by seeming to avoid any wrongdoing. It is our contention that this higher standard is appropriately applied to psychiatrists, and that such a standard illustrates the distinctiveness of psychiatric ethics. Because psychiatrists must undertake these societal duties on which public trust is so reliant, they will be required to go beyond ordinary virtue,

---

[12] Without that knowledge, citizens must judge "presumptively" in Dennis Thompson's term, in concluding that a large contribution from an interested party is *likely* to function as a bribe (in the case of the legislator). Elected representatives must thus avoid acting under conditions that give rise to a reasonable belief of wrongdoing. When they fail to do so, they fall from the high ethical standard required by their role and, as Thompson puts it, "they do not merely appear to do wrong, they do wrong" (Thompson 1995: 126).

and certainly ordinary moral rules. Demands such as these that go beyond duty (or ordinary virtue) are sometimes described as "supererogatory" (See Heyd, 2006).

If psychiatrists are to avoid the appearance of wrongdoing in addition to avoiding wrongdoing itself, we argue in Chapter 5, they must cultivate what we are naming the virtue of propriety or carefulness over appearances. The kind of concern for appearances, or propriety, that we are proposing is illustrated by the following case.

> Dr. A, a psychiatrist, was married to a psychologist (Dr. B) whose expertise lay in dealing with patients in abusive relationships. Because of this expertise, Dr. A believed a referral of his patient's abusive husband to Dr. B would be justified. However, he decided to refer his patient's husband elsewhere lest the referral to his own wife appear questionable due to the "double" financial benefit to the practitioners involved.

Here, Dr. A exhibited a sensitivity to appearances, and refrained from making the referral not because it would compromise him ethically, but because it would appear to do so. Notice, then, that his response was a role-constituted one. In everyday life we rarely find it necessary to adhere to, or ask for, the appearance of ethical behavior in addition to ethical behavior itself—we just demand (of ourselves and others) ethical behavior. The extra demand, here, was imposed by Dr. A's role.

The need for extra virtue, and for this particular, role-constituted (supererogatory) virtue of propriety, illustrates the particular aptness of virtue ethics in this context. Demands that cannot be universalized present a greater problem for other ethical frameworks, and can readily be accommodated within virtue ethics. To illustrate: criticism leveled at the appearance standard applied to public officials insisting that it contravenes principles fundamental to our legal system indicates how this is so. To impose professional censure on a person (an official, a practitioner) only guilty of the appearance of wrongdoing, it has been objected, seems to be to prejudge the facts, perhaps to impose retroactive rules, and to censure a blameless person (Stark 1995). This critique can arise, we suggest, only because of the deontological underpinnings of those legal principles. The extra virtue or virtues required by the practitioner's role may be particular, and not "universalizable" in their scope, presenting themselves as character ideals to be striven after, rather than duties. Care over appearances is called for by features of the professional setting. But it is better understood as a virtue to be cultivated, we maintain, than a rule to be followed. When this focus on appearances is thus in the form of an ideal, rather than a rule, and applies only to the practitioner within the professional role, these criticisms of appearance standards have little remaining force.

Further aspects of the psychiatry setting seem to call for such supererogatory virtues. Several critics have enunciated the dangers in managed medical care and the bureaucratized, segmented medical delivery systems of today: some of these criticisms even employ virtue language. One of these critiques, by Frank Chervenak and Laurence McCullough (2001), shows another place where the practitioner must go above and beyond rules and duties.

These authors focus their attention on the moral leadership required now that institutions play a central role in medical care. Because individual physicians discharge their fiduciary obligations in and through institutions, they note "Physician-leaders, more than individual physicians in practice, bear the responsibility to shape organizations' cultures that support the fiduciary professionalism of physicians with daily responsibility for patient care, medical education and research" (Chervenak and McCullough 2001: 879). Managed care medicine requires several traits until now not required of doctors. Only with a combination of managerial and moral excellence, the latter acquired through the cultivation of particular virtues, will doctors fulfill a leadership role in these organizations. (We will return to the particular virtues endorsed by these authors in a later discussion.)

Notice some of the implicit reasoning that draws Chervenak and McCullough's argument along. The economic goals of managed care organizations seem to be orthogonal, if not outright antithetical, to the professional goals of physicians, which entail a fiduciary relationship with patients. Because of that, and because these new arrangements force them to work within systems directed toward these economic goals, physicians will need to cultivate the particular moral virtues to equip them for moral, medical leadership. Yet the demand for leadership, by its nature, goes beyond duty. A leader is exceptional, a remarkable character, whose traits enable the accomplishment of feats beyond the capabilities of many others, and so beyond what could be required of everyone. A deontological ethical system offers moral rules that apply to all. To capture the unique moral heights achieved by, and the demands that can be made of, a leader, we are better served by the flexibility and idiosyncratic notions of virtues and individual character. (In addition to this demand for moral leadership, today's bureaucratized care delivery systems require other special virtues, and these are introduced in Chapter 5.)

Conclusion

A virtue ethics framework, we showed in this chapter, has particular applicability to the practice of psychiatry. In addition, it suits the role morality associated with all professionals and seems to comport well with features common to all medical practice. So a focus on virtues, and on the character of the practitioner, will be appropriate to psychiatric practice for the same reasons that it is to any medical practice, and also to any professional practice.

The particular advantages provided by the virtue-based approach were shown to include its acknowledgment of inner states as well as outer responses; its provision of a more complete moral psychology; its allowance for the "unruly" affective nature of many virtues and especially those called for by the doctor–patient relationship; and its accommodation of a "partial" rather than "impartial" attitude toward moral demands. Over and above that, we drew attention to features of the psychiatry setting that further explain why a virtue ethics framework seems to fit psychiatric practice. First, aspects of the interpersonal relationship essential to effective practice seem to call for a number of affective responses not subject to immediate control and thus not conducive to a focus on rules. These unruly responses are only reliably manifested as the result of the process of habituation involved in the cultivation of virtues. Second, the particular social roles and responsibilities imposed on the psychiatrist demand something beyond dutiful behavior. In not only avoiding wrongdoing, but appearing to avoid wrongdoing, practitioners exceed what could be deemed their duty, in deontological terms, that is, universalizable rules of conduct. And this demand is best understood in terms of the possession of special virtue and of special and additional virtues. Finally, we saw that the need for particular virtues required by today's care delivery systems seems to be magnified in the psychiatry setting. One virtue called for by that setting is the supererogatory traits associated with the moral leadership required to defend the fiduciary goals of medicine.

In Chapter 5, we explore the character of the virtuous psychiatrist more fully, examining what kind of traits role constituted virtues are, their particular moral and psychological ingredients, their allied temptations or vices, and the aspects of the psychiatry setting to which they are responses. Before that, however, we must look at the systemic effect of gender on every aspect of the practice setting. In Chapter 4, we outline these effects and their implications for psychiatric ethics and the character and moral psychology of the virtuous psychiatrist.

4 Elements of a Gender-Sensitive Ethics for Psychiatry

From a feminist perspective it might seem self-evident that therapeutic relationships, like all relationships, would be fundamentally constituted by the gender of the participants.

CAROLYN QUADRIO (2001: 121)

Introduction

The term "gender" is confusingly ambiguous: sometimes it is used to include and sometimes to exclude the biological bases of sexual assignment. When sex and gender are counterpoised, sex refers to the biologically "given" (vagina, ovaries, DNA, for example) while gender, in contrast, refers to the culturally shaped attributes of femininity and masculinity associated with gender role and gender identity. In our discussion, gender encompasses not only biological traits but culturally wrought attributes as well.

Understood that way, gender has a special place in psychiatry, and psychiatry's practitioners seem likely required to cultivate gender-sensitive virtues for at least two reasons. First, because of the centrality of gender as a category in our culture and the nature of the healing project in psychiatry, gender identity will be an almost inescapable ingredient in that project. Second, gender has been entwined with norms of mental health throughout Western history, and psychiatric theory, lore, and practice have for so long been imbued with assumptions and presuppositions about gender that they can hardly fail to reflect them still. Indeed, psychiatric theory and practice are "gendered" as, arguably, are no other medical subspecialties except those directly involved with dimorphic traits (obstetrics, gynecology, and urology, for example). There are gender-linked disorders and evidence of gender-linked treatment differences; gendering appears in diagnostic categories and classifications, in theories of development and norms of mental health, in associations and cultural tropes pertinent to psychiatry, and in the everyday language without which treatment could not be conducted. All these, together with healing practices that are the systemic effects of our society's past "masculinist" traditions, such as centuries of the treatment of women patients by men practitioners, have influenced one another and in turn served to shape the psychiatric theory and lore that guide practice even today.

Like gender, race, class, and ethnicity also contribute to—or "constitute"—people's identities. And other cultural and political categories such as race, class, and ethnicity are also implicated in the normative presuppositions of psychiatry (Fabrega 1990, 1991; Nissim-Sabat 2004). So in that respect, we can see gender as one of several kinds of framing elements central to practice. Moreover, gender intersects with these other elements. The Aristotelian Table of Opposites introduces the underlying value dichotomy system of which our traditional notions of gender are a legacy. There, Nancy Potter reminds us, "light" is on the side of "goodness" and "maleness," while "dark" is located in the column along with "female" and "evil." Thus although the asymmetrical value system that perpetuates gender inferiority for women and gender superiority for men has been far reaching in its effects for both women and men, the racial axis of power complicates this analysis even further. People of color—both men and women—are often characterized in ways similar to the qualities associated with femaleness, such as emotionality, Potter explains. So "any thoroughgoing understanding of gender as a contributor to mental ease or distress must include considerations of racialization processes and experiences of being raced" (Potter 2004: 239).

Attention in the present book is limited to gender but we recognize the interconnections just noted. Gender is one, particularly notable, example of the way psychiatry is a practice embedded in culture. Although not possible here, a more complete analysis would include racial, ethnic, and class differences, and their interaction with gender, as well.

As was noted at the outset, sex and gender are sometimes counterpoised. "Sex" refers to biological characteristics and "gender" to the nonbiological, culturally shaped attributes associated with the styles and traits known as femininity and masculinity. Although useful as a rough guide, this distinction is not, finally, a viable one and will not be relied upon here. Its underlying assumption that biological attributes are immutable givens and not shaped by culture is unsustainable, as we hope the following chapter will illustrate.

In addition to the misleading binary thinking underlying the distinction often drawn between sex and gender, we will explore some other dualistic presuppositions often associated with it. One of these is the presumption that normally there are but two sexes and two corresponding (normal) genders. Another is the assumption, also widely accepted in our culture, that a person's biological and culturally shaped gender attributes are equally fixed and immutable, remaining unchanged through that person's lifetime. These presuppositions in turn underlie traditional conceptions of normal gender identity, the self-ascribed gender attributes of the person.

Rather than rejecting—or indeed, endorsing—this set of distinctions, assumptions, and presuppositions (sex/gender; masculine/feminine; male/female) we want to emphasize the uncertainties and controversies surrounding each of them. Because these underlying assumptions and presuppositions are contested, we argue, ethical constraints are imposed on the practitioner in psychiatry: in particular, certain gender-sensitive responses are required of those entrusted to engage with questions of gender identity. This is not to assert that such presuppositions cannot reflect universal truths. Rather, it is to emphasize that they have the status of hypotheses, whose validity remains uncertain.

The focus and positions adopted in this discussion require a further word of explanation. First, we recognize that the ethical issues implicating gender are more numerous than those discussed here. (One of these other issues, sexual exploitation by the practitioner, has been introduced already and is raised briefly at the end of this chapter.) We have elected to explore the ethical issues surrounding gender identity more fully at the expense of other matters for several reasons. As was noted above, gender identity here constitutes a particularly important example of identity characterizations based on status (such as race, ethnicity, or class). Moreover, an unprecedented new emphasis on self-defined identity of this kind has been the result of identity politics. Questions of identity in this sense of self-characterization are inescapable in cultures such as ours. Part and parcel of identity politics, however, is a particular liberal-democratic ideology that assigns the subject unprecedented power over her (characterization) identity. (In political theorizing, this is portrayed as an individual [and group] "liberty right"—the right to "recognition," and associated with the work of thinkers like Charles Taylor, and Nancy Fraser, introduced earlier.) This powerful and pervasive set of values, widely shared, also has strong echoes in bioethics, where individual autonomy is frequently treated not as the sole, but as the primary, and as the presumptive or "default," value.

Within this complex and politicized arena, the position adopted by the ethical practitioner must be a delicate one. The ideology that places the assignment of gender identity in the hands of the subject may not be shared, and need not be adopted or endorsed by the practitioner. (The practitioner may adhere to more traditional ideas about gender norms, for example.) Because of the controversy surrounding such ideology, combined with the presumption, from identity politics and bioethics, that accords to the (competent) individual autonomy over gender identity, however, the practitioner's task may be to assist in the patient's exploration of the underlying experiences, values, ideas, and ideals—and ultimately, the patient's conception of the good life—that ground her self-assigned gender identity. In the context where patients suffer severe mental disorder, this approach will not always—and may not often—be possible, it is true. When delusional thinking interferes, for example, the patient's assessment of her own gender identity cannot be approached, and honored, this way. Nor can it be accepted if accompanied by what are patently self-destructive impulses, or the intention to harm others. Yet even in the absence of such disqualifying symptoms, and in light of present day political realities and of the controversy surrounding questions of gender (outlined in this chapter), it is difficult to avoid the conclusion that, like the rest of bioethics, within psychiatry, individual autonomy must be the default value guiding practice.

This chapter is laid out in the following way. We begin by exploring the notion of gender identity. Whatever that identity may be, because of the centrality of gender to identity, the patient's gender identity is an inescapable factor in treatment and in the therapeutic project. We emphasize the need for acknowledgment and recognition of the centrality of gender identity by the practitioner. We then turn to six key ways in which psychiatry appears to be a complexly "gendered" practice. These include epidemiological findings that correlate one gender or another with particular disorders; the evidence of "gendering" in certain diagnostic categories and symptom descriptions; an observed gender link in treatment variations; the presence of gendering in normative theories and lore about mental health; the cultural tropes and associations assigning mental disorder to women and the feminine; and finally, the gendering of the everyday language in which all psychiatric treatment is conducted. We then explore some of the implications of practicing psychiatry within a gender conscious and gender-biased society with a legacy of masculinist traditions. We also emphasize the uncertainty and controversy attaching to each of the several binary distinctions underlying traditional thinking about gender; such uncertainty and controversy seem to require that the ethical practitioner reflect on gender. And finally, we pursue these conclusions in relation to the responses required of the gender-sensitive practitioner.

Gender Identity

In our culture, at least, gender plays a constitutive role in identity forma-tion and construction. As the aspect of one's self-concept or characterization identity that relates to one's own gender, gender identity is interwoven with three elements. (Characterization identity, as was noted earlier, concerns not the metaphysical self or personal identity in the deepest philosophical sense, but the socially constructed self-concept.) First is gender attribution by others, the complex interactive process of inferring and then attributing the gender of someone on the basis of the observable features, such as clothing, that func-tion as gender signifiers. Second is the special case of gender attribution made at birth and usually based on an inspection of the infant's genitals, known as gender assignment. And finally, there is gender role, the set of prescriptions and expectations believed appropriate for each gender.

Because of its contribution to identity (in our culture, at least), gender cannot but be part of the psychiatric project. This may not be so everywhere. We know there are cultures in which the gender divide differs in its details, is more forgivingly blurred, or is less socially salient. Ethnologists do not always agree on how other cultures' variations on our dichotomous gender system are to be classified (Ramet 1996). But they describe several cultures including Native American ones in which an apparent third gender, or "ber-dache," is acknowledged and socially sanctioned (Goulet 2001); they point to the category of Hijras in India, which is made up of transsexuals, effemi-nate men, and eunuchs (Nanda 1989); and they note cultures such as that of the Yoruba in which age seems to replace gender as the salient stratifying category (Oyewumi 1997). In our culture though, it seems impossible for us to envision a person's self-concept or characterization identity without some gender assignment—even if it is something unusual, such as "masculine and feminine," or "mixed," or "in between," or even "alternating."

The goal of therapy may be understood in terms of an ideal of mental health that acknowledges traditional binary gendering (there are two normal genders that remain fixed, so everyone either strives to be a mentally healthy man or a mentally healthy woman). Alternatively, it may be understood in terms of some variant on that: one strives to be a mentally healthy transgendered, "bigendered,"[1] or intersexed person or a mentally healthy androgynous person. But whichever conception is employed in the way the therapeutic project is defined, conceptions of gender will be integral to the therapeutic process and to the criteria by which progress is assessed.

Epidemiology

Enshrined in research methodology, the categories and presuppositions associated with gender are also inescapably tied to psychiatry through epidemiology. Inquiry into the incidence and course of disorders with an eye to identifying gender patterns has been part of Western medicine from its beginnings. Gender links with disorders such as melancholia were frequently hazarded, although for the most part premodern estimates are transparently confounded by their misogynist assumptions (Hirshbein 2006; Lunbeck 1994; Radden 2000; Showalter 1986). Strong gender links with eating disorder have been established more recently, placing such disorder as the most frequently diagnosed mental disorder in young women today (Crandall 2004; Zalta and Keel 2006). Certain personality disorders, such as Antisocial Personality Disorder, are similarly gender linked to men (APA 1994: 631–632).

In acknowledgment of both biological and of cultural differences between women and men, gender has been seen as a research category of fundamental importance, and recent evidence on several mental disorders reveals gender links in incidence, as well as such factors as age of onset, course, and response to therapy. Thus, for example, the findings with regard to depression indicate not only that women are more prone to depression but that they are more likely than men to have a first onset of depression during adolescence, will more often than men develop rapid cycling bipolar conditions, and will respond differently to a range of different treatments (Frank 2000; Kaplan and Sadock 1995).

---

[1] Being "bigendered" is understood from time to time as switching between masculine and feminine gender roles.

Although it is widely reported that women show a greater incidence of affective disorder, gender links in the incidence of mental disorder diagnoses overall are more difficult to read. They are confused by inconsistent definitions of mental disorder and real disagreement over its boundaries. When the substance abuse and personality disorders previously regarded as deviance rather than illness were categorized with traditional disorders such as depression and schizophrenia, a surprisingly even distribution of mental disorder among men and women emerged (Kessler et al. 1994; Prior 1999; Robins and Regier 1991). The debate over the inclusion of these kinds of problem associated with men in definitions of mental illness may itself reflect presuppositions about gender. Within a health care structure dominated by patriarchal values and ideals, as Pauline Prior observes, it had long been "easier to define the problems of women as illness and those of men as deviance. . . . In this way, the macho image of the 'strong' man and the 'weak' woman was maintained" (Prior 1999: 47).

Diagnostic Categories

Of the several ways in which psychiatric practice is gendered in Western nosologies perhaps most familiar are gender-specific disorders such as Homosexuality, Gender Identity Disorder, Premenstrual Dysphoric Disorder, and other gender-biased diagnostic categories (Caplan 1995a, 1995b; Prior 1999: 93; Sadler 2005).[2] Reference has already been made to hysteria and homosexuality as diagnostic categories, but gender bias has also been attributed to classifications such as Dependent Personality Disorder, Self-Defeating Personality Disorder, and Histrionic Personality Disorder (Sadler 2005; Widiger and Spitzer 1991). Other critics have drawn attention to the apparent protection from psychiatric classification—through "normalizing"—of male responses and behavioral patterns (Caplan 1995a: 168–173); moreover, although homosexuality is no longer regarded as a disorder as such, current diagnoses identify children "growing up gay" as pathological (Isay 1997; Richardson et al. 1999). And while homosexuality, and even ego-dystonic homosexuality, have been expunged from the most recent DSM, there remains a

---

[2] In non-Western and particularly Asian settings, the common condition of "koro" or genital retraction delusions are another case of gendered disorder (Chowdhury 1998).

condition entitled "Persistent and marked distress about sexual orientation" (APA 1994: 538).[3] (See Sadler 2005; Soble 2004.)

One Controversial Diagnostic Category: Gender Identity Disorder

The category of Gender Identity Disorder (GID) was introduced at the outset of this work: it is emblematic of the way psychiatry is entwined with cultural norms. GID has been shown to entail a collection of particularly controversial presuppositions about gender and, as an increasingly common diagnosis, it deserves special attention. Centered on precisely the contrast often drawn between sex and gender, this diagnostic category finds disturbance in patients' characterization of themselves as possessed of a gender at odds with their biological traits: it has been defined as "a strong and persistent cross-gender identification accompanied by a persistent discomfort with one's assigned sex" (APA 1994: 532–533).

Several of the most trenchant criticisms of this disorder category rest on its reliance on apparently arbitrary, socially constructed categories and norms, particularly the strict gender dualism asserting that male and female, masculine and feminine are exhaustive categories and that every individual's sex, gender, and sexuality are natural, singular, and invariant across his or her life. (See also Feder 1997; Morgan 2002; Nelson 2001; Scheman 1997.) In the words of one of these critics, GID is a classification that serves to reinforce, and legitimate, controversial and contested social norms with regard to masculinity and femininity (Feder, 1997).

Others have taken issue with the suggestion that discomfort with and suffering over one's gender identity constitutes an indicator of GID. They point out that if such discomfort stems from the enforcement of arbitrary societal norms or "gender policing," to use Katherine Morgan's vivid term, and particularly from the presumption that the biologically given and constructed aspects of one's gender must comport with one another, then this involves circular reasoning. Societal norms require these people to present themselves in ways that contradict how they feel, and then pathologize their condition based on the discomfort that dissonance produces. (See Morgan 2002.)[4] The DSM offers a criterion for distinguishing "endogenous," from merely social-engendered "exogamous" distress over sexual fantasies, urges,

---

[3] This appears under Sexual Disorders Not Otherwise Specified.

[4] Signs of a reconsideration of these approaches to "intersex" conditions are now found. See, for example, Frader et al. (2004).

or behavior. But as Alan Soble has pointed out, any disorder status reliant upon the DSM category of "endogenous" distress will be difficult to employ in all cases (Soble 2004).

Recently, some transsexuals portrayed as suffering from GID have come to see themselves as victims of, rather than appropriately fitting, that diagnosis. They support the concept of an encompassing "transgenderism," which draws in all "gender-variant" identities and asks recognition of diverse sexual beings within the realm of healthy normalcy, including those whose bodies seem at odds with their preferred gender roles and gender identity. In transgenderism the once-emphasized distinction between transsexuals and transvestites, for example, is "supplanted . . . with a concept of continuity" (Bolin 1994: 461); moreover, in contrast to their earlier goal of crossing from one traditional gender identity to another through sex reassignment treatment, today's transsexuals increasingly seek to maintain a transgendered identity that is neither male nor female in the traditional sense. (See Atkins 1998; Borstein 1994; Feinberg 1996, 1998.)

Gendered Treatment Variations

Past studies have indicated that women receive different treatments from men. Thus at least in the 1980s it was shown that women receive more drug treatment in all classes of drugs, with the greatest difference in psychotropic drugs (Cooperstock 1981). Throughout Europe and the United States, women were prescribed approximately twice as many psychotropic drugs per head as men (Ashton 1991), as they were in Australia during the same period (Quadrio 2001). Again in studies dating from this period, evidence suggested that male doctors were more likely to perceive physical complaints as psychological disorder when the patient was a woman (Ashton 1991). Other studies showed women less likely than men to be referred on from primary care providers to mental health specialists (Shapiro 1990; Vehaak 1993). Whether these forms of bias have been reduced as the result of awareness of them, and as increased numbers of women have entered the specialty, awaits further study.

Normative Theories and Lore

Normative theories and lore about mental health also represent a central strand of psychiatric thinking and practice. Many of these stem from the psychoanalytic theorizing of Freud and his followers in the first half of the twentieth century, which accepted the binary systems noted earlier of male and female, masculine and feminine. Because of the biological and cultural differences between males and females, the achievement of mature adjustment was seen as reached through very different developmental paths, and as comprising separate roles and satisfactions for men and women, respectively (Freud 1959). "Separate" proved not to be equal, however. Studies conducted in the 1960s and 1970s revealed reliance on a pervasive evaluative dualism by which the norms of mental health were male and masculine (Broverman et al. 1970; Maccoby 1998). By the middle of the twentieth century, as well, these norms came to be associated with gender orthodoxy, especially conventional gender roles, heterosexuality, and marriage; to contravene such norms was to exhibit pathology (Bem 1995; Connell 1995).

Also tracing to psychoanalytic theorizing are notions pertaining to the degree of autonomy found in the healthy self. By favoring individualistic models of independence and autonomy that are associated with male socialization and masculinity, such thinking has been judged as not only a politicized ideal favoring individualistic rather than more collectivist or communitarian models, but a gendered one. Such norms have been criticized as positing a conception of self not even realistic, let alone desirable, and particularly unfitting to women's socialization and gender identity (Card 1991; Christman 2004; Christman and Anderson 2006; Meyers 1997; Radden 1996; Richardson et al. 1999).

Cultural Tropes and Associations

Historians have argued that several widely accepted presuppositions about gender, including the assigning of homosexuality to immature, and or maladaptive, status, are of relatively recent origin. The classification of homosexuality as unhealthy has been dated to the nineteenth century, for example (Katz 1990, 1995). Coming of age during the era when homosexuality was regarded as contrary to norms of mental health, as modern psychiatry did, we should not be surprised that this set of presumptions about what constituted healthy sexual development and behavior became entrenched in psychiatric thinking.

But not all the gendering we find in modern psychiatry stems from such recent times. Gender, understood in the broad way employed here (including biological as well as cultural attributes) is tied to practice through cultural tropes and associations that go back to the beginnings of Western thought and medical practice. The central categories within which mental disorder has been understood in our traditions—rationality and the reasoning capacities, the passions, the mind, beliefs, moods, emotions, the will, the self and self-control—were all, for hundreds of years, strongly associated with one sex or another, or gendered (Lloyd 1993). Historically and in more recent times, psychiatric categories, diagnoses, treatment, and research have reflected these associations. Like madness itself, the feminine connoted irrationality, unbridled passion, immaturity, the bodily, and carnality, linking the feminine with disorder by powerful strands of cultural influence (Busfield 1986, 1996; Potter 2004; Russell 1994; Showalter 1986; Skultans 1979; Ussher 1991; Wenegrat 1995).

The once-common diagnostic category of hysteria, with its female and feminine connotations, is only the most obvious example of these strands. Another example is to be found in the associations, confirmed in subsequent epidemiology, linking women with depression and other mood disorders. The broad category of melancholia had since classical times enjoyed associations of brilliance and creativity, tying it to maleness. However, eighteenth and nineteenth century faculty psychology firmly separated the cognitive from the affective, so that by the beginnings of modern psychiatry the affective was associated with what were deemed women's traits—capriciousness, uncontrolled emotionality, irrationality, the bodily, and the subjective. Women's bodies, particularly, with their distinctive reproductive features and phases, were thought to render women vulnerable to disorders of affect. And by the last decades of the nineteenth century, asylum records were supporting a strong gender link between women and the affective conditions Kraepelin entitled manic depression (Lunbeck 1994; Radden 2000: 39–44; Showalter 1986).

If for no other reason, this long cultural legacy in which madness and its seat in the mental faculties were all gendered categories means that the question of gender is unavoidable in any discussion of mental health norms and care, and it demands the attention accorded it in this volume.

Language

Gender presuppositions are to be found not only in our behavior, beliefs, and attitudes but in spoken language, the communicative vehicle of almost all healing practice in psychiatry. Earlier work on nonsexist and gender-sensitive doctor–patient relationships, emphasized that derogatory and demeaning labels must be avoided. (See, for example, Bishop 1992.) But this may not be sufficient. Gender differences are "marked and constituted, in part, by the words we utter and the kind of speech acts we engage in," as Potter puts it (Potter 2004: 241). One example will suffice here: in ordinary language the term "work" has customarily been restricted to wage labor undertaken away from home. The effect of this definition, which allows assertions such as "She doesn't work; she's home with the kids" immediately precludes recognition of many forms of important, arduous, unpaid domestic effort traditionally undertaken by women. Given the respect accorded work in our culture, the effect of this linguistic pattern in reinforcing masculinist attitudes and values is evident.

If, as has been insisted, the very structure and components of language itself privilege males and masculinity, then nothing less than an alternative discourse may be required for those who are nonmales or unmasculine, or both, which, unlike the dominant discourse, will allow them to better recognize and express themselves as subjects (Irigaray 1985). We return to this issue of language later in this chapter as we explore the responses appropriate to a gender-sensitive practitioner.

Practicing Psychiatry Within Masculinist (Patriarchal) Cultural Traditions

Finally, it has been pointed out that gender is central to psychiatry because such practice takes place within a culture that has long been systematically masculinist or "patriarchal." This will be no less true for any other medical or indeed any other professional practice, yet it still requires acknowledgment. The division between women's and men's roles has long brought power differentials. These differentials are reinforced by what has been at least until very recently the typical encounter where the female patient is cared for by a male practitioner, with each enacting culturally entrenched roles and power dynamics—those of powerless help-seeker and powerful expert/patriarchal healer, in Laura Brown's words (Brown 1994). Not only race, ethnicity, and class, as we noted earlier, but sexual orientation, age, and disability function interactively with gender in "overlapping and recursive ways," Brown points out, and with their various signifiers can lend special meaning to each person in the interaction, with profound effects on "how power is experienced and shared in the therapeutic context." (Brown 1994: 98–99) This factor has also been emphasized by others (Busfield 1996; Dunn 1998; Karasu 1999). Because they are accustomed to systemic power imbalances in other parts of their lives—and especially so, perhaps, if they are also poor or non-white—women in this situation will experience their power as reduced and diminished to a greater degree than would those not so culturally positioned. When replicating within the therapeutic relationship the power arrangement in which women traditionally found and still find themselves in the broader society, psychiatry as a practice must be particularly attentive to not perpetuating unjust social and cultural patterns. And individual straight, male practitioners working with patients who are neither, have particular ethical obligations.

Gender as Controversial

Uncertainty and controversy attach to traditional presuppositions about gender in at least three fundamental dimensions. The distinction underlying the sex/gender contrast, between biologically fixed and culturally formed, has been challenged by thinkers such as Anne Fausto-Sterling. Fausto-Sterling points out that, for example, the standard practice of surgically correcting sexually ambiguous infants to render them unambiguously male or female represents a cultural intervention. The interplay between apparently biologically given and culturally constructed here blurs any sex/gender distinction because, as she puts it, "it is possible to visualize the medical and biological only by peering through a cultural screen" (Fausto-Sterling 2000: 95).

Also challenged in recent years, as we have seen, has been the presupposition that there are only two normal, healthy genders. Not only does this binary thinking appear to be historically recent, and at odds with the diversity of gender roles and identities evident in some other cultures, but the biological evidence indicates the presence of a spectrum of intermediate, intersexed cases between fully biologically female and biologically male. Emphasizing the presence of biological variability, one radical proposal would add three more categories to the categories of female and male, thus expanding the types of normal, healthy gender from two to five by including true hermaphrodites, and male and female pseudohermaphrodites (Fausto-Sterling 2000: 101). This proposal illustrates the extent of the controversy surrounding traditional presuppositions about gender.

Finally, the assumption that normal gender identity is always unchanged throughout the lifetime of the person has recently been questioned. The very term "identity" in the notion of gender identity hints that one's gender is fixed early, and thereafter immutable (although not always recognized to be so). Yet historians and anthropologists remind us of cultures in which developmental stages are associated with alternative sexual behavior and gender roles. (In classical Greece, adolescent males engaged in genital acts with older men; later, they married and adopted "heterosexuality.") Some anecdotal evidence, and the better known cases of the gender preference of bisexuality, manifested serially, suggest that not merely developmental stages but adult life phases may give rise to different gender preferences and proclivities. Different genders and gender identities may occur in one person within the course of that person's lifetime. This alternative, too, can—and some theorists propose should—be reconstrued as normal variation within the range of healthy possibilities.

We note these growing controversies around gender, it should again be emphasized, not to adopt one position or another but in order to provide the grounds for our insistence that an ethical practitioner in psychiatry must be gender sensitive.

Gender-Sensitive Practice

A characterization of gender-sensitive virtues will be more fully developed in the chapter following this one. The first step towards that end, however, requires us to acknowledge the complex way gender is woven throughout psychiatric theory and practice and the range of controversies gender categories have invited, exploring the behavioral, communicative, and attitudinal responses these investigations call for. Present day voices about gender, from scholars, theorists, and activists, are remarkably discordant. But a handful of commonalities, seemingly agreed-upon by many, have emerged out of the tumult, and even these invite particular ethical responses from practitioners. (Some of these commonalities are very obvious, and suggest responses long prescribed and practiced within psychiatry, but in order to prepare for our later discussion of gender-sensitive professional's virtues for the practitioner, they, too, must be included in what follows.)

Agreed-upon are as follows: (i) gender is a central category in our culture; (ii) the consequent significance of gender for self or characterization identity; (iii) many strands of gender partiality are built into psychiatric theory, lore, and practice; (iv) within a broader masculinist/patriarchal cultural setting like ours there are power dimensions that affect practices such as psychiatry; (v) controversy surrounds most if not all traditional gender assumptions; and finally, (vi) rightly or wrongly, transgender and other activists have sought to define their own gender identity.

The centrality and importance of gender in our culture and the consequent significance of gender to identity are matters to which the ethical practitioner must respond with attention and imagination. First, attention: gender cannot be ignored. In emphasizing that we seek gender-sensitive responses in the practitioner here, we want to avoid gender blind ones. Writing about gender ideals in education, Jane Martin has observed that in a society where traits are gendered and socialization according to sex is a commonplace, trying to ignore gender in the name of equality reinforces the stereotypes and unequal practices it claims to abhor, "making invisible the problems it should be addressing." Gender sensitivity, according to Martin, requires us to be "constantly aware of the workings of sex and gender" (Martin 1985: 195).

So to imagination: the "constant awareness" involved in the gender sensitivity recommended here, we want to emphasize, must include an empathic and imaginative exploration of the patient's own presuppositions about gender and gender identity. Rather than merely discovering, or observing that identity, the ethical practitioner will explore its meaning in relation to the rest of the self, the way it feels, and the attitudes it engenders. This will not always, and perhaps not often, be possible, as we saw earlier, because gender identity may be distorted by delusional thinking. But when it is possible, the patient can be helped to see the experiences, values, ideas, and ideals undergirding the formation of her gender identity. Moreover, this will not be a single or closed inquiry, but rather an open-ended and ongoing alertness to the element of gender in the patient's identity and experience.

Even with such attitudes of awareness habituated in character, how must the practitioner position herself and her own attitudes in relation to the patient's gender identity? One starting point for this discussion might be the "International Bill of Gender Rights" put forward by transgender activists (IBGR 1995). Employing the language and strategies of all liberation and identity politics, this document includes a right to "define gender identity" (as well as to control and change one's own body). Transgender activists may avoid the mental health care setting, if only to be free to exercise this right. Yet, their plea to decide for themselves how their own personal gender will be delineated is one that, if legitimate, would have application within psychiatric practice. The practitioner who honors this demand rather than imposing a gender identity on the patient will allow the patient to define where she fits within the spectrum of gender assignments, as well as how she evaluates her identity—as healthy or unhealthy, shameful or acceptable, valid or troubling.

> Dr. K's patient, a successful, articulate, 28-year-old male lawyer, came to the point immediately: he had begun hormonal treatment for a male to female sex reassignment and before his planned surgery, required a letter from a psychiatrist confirming that the condition was long-standing. He had always known something was wrong, he explained to Dr. K, and on reaching adulthood concluded that he was really a woman, trapped in an increasingly abhorrent male body.

Further inquiry may not confirm this patient's claims. But if it does, then seemingly—unless Dr. K took the patient to be delusional or recognized other psychopathology—Dr. K may be required to honor the patient's request.

The caveats are of course critical. Few rights, however protected, can be exercised without certain basic cognitive and communicative capabilities, the capabilities frequently compromised by severe mental disorder. Such disorder can generate delusions as to gender identity, for example.[5] And the practitioner who honored this alleged right (to define one's own gender identity) for an identity reliant on delusional thinking, would fail her patient. When the basic cognitive and communicative capabilities required for rights are present, however, and the patient's gender identity is not apparently based on delusion, or likely to be immediately self-destructive or harmful to others, the right to define one's own gender identity should perhaps be accepted. Why honor such a right? Merely, we suggested earlier, because of the controversy we have seen surrounding the concept of gender, the culture-wide recognition of the importance of self-defined identity, and, within bioethics, the default or presumptive honoring of individual autonomy.

To emphasize the right to transgress traditional ideas and ideals about gender is hardly the only, or even perhaps the most important, lesson to be learned from the indisputable claims in points discussed from (i) to (vi)

---

[5] For a classic description, see Daniel Paul Schreber's account of his delusions.

above. Rather than challenging traditional presuppositions about gender, most people in our culture accept them, often with a conviction which, in light of the controversy those presuppositions have given rise to in recent years, may be misplaced. Still widely assumed, and often endorsed, is the belief that male and female, masculine and feminine, are exhaustive categories and the associated view that every individual's sex, gender, and sexuality are natural, singular, and invariant across his or her life.

The controversy attaching to each of these beliefs also calls for particular ethical responses from the practitioner. However attached to these ideas and ideals the practitioner may be personally, he or she must recognize as undeniable the extent to which our gender norms are controversial and unresolved. This is not to claim that any such beliefs about gender are merely subjective, or absolutely right, but only that the status of such claims is uncertain. This recognition in turn will—or should—yield tolerance. For the ethical practitioner who acknowledges the status of her own beliefs, tolerance of other practices and norms and other forms of gender identity can be the only stance to adopt.[6] This acknowledgment will, or should, also yield humility. The practitioner who is aware of the controversy surrounding gender must conclude that his or her own particular set of beliefs, theories, and attitudes about gender likely contain at least some misapprehensions, parochial prejudices, and unwarranted assumptions. Because like other forms of self-characterization or characterization identity, gender identity is increasingly recognized to be idiosyncratic, self-defined, and arbitrary, the ethical psychiatrist will need to possess the empathic understanding we associate with the imagination.

The response of the informed and ethical practitioner in this setting is complex. She knows at once too much and too little about gender. She must recognize, avoid, and sometimes even interpret to the patient the harmful gendering implicit in aspects of psychiatric theory, lore, and practice, as well as in the very language in which the therapeutic exchange is conducted. But she must also acknowledge the controversial and uncertain status of claims about gender and adopt, and convey, the appropriate stance in the face of such uncertainty.

---

[6] The perspective we are proposing here is akin to the more general epistemological position known as standpoint theory, adopted by many feminists. See, for example, Mahowald (1996).

Should the ethical practitioner at least have worked out her own account of gender, which could guide some of her practice decisions and goals? We believe not. Take just one aspect of such an account, the relation of gender to norms of mental health and the issue of androgyny. (See Elshtain 1987; Ferguson 1977; Garber 1996; Heilbrun 1980; Weil 1992.) In psychiatric practice, androgynous ideals have somewhat replaced earlier sex-specific mental health norms. Women too, it has been emphasized, can be assertive, competent, logical, and self-controlled, and these traits can be reconstrued so that they are understood as gender neutral. Moreover, in recognition of "cultural feminism" there have been efforts to revive, reclaim, and valorize appreciation of long denigrated feminine traits such as emotionality. (See Gilligan 1982; Jordan et al. 1991; Miller 1976; Miller and Stiver 1998; Robb 2007.) At the same time, findings about biological differences between the sexes, including several in brain structure and function, have led to an emphasis on differentiated norms (Legato 2004; Peplau 2003; Vawter et al 2004; Wager et al 2003). And it has also been proposed that gender is not merely as an attribute of individual personality and self-identity but as an emergent property of social groups, the product of biological predispositions that, varying between the (two) sexes, have in turn stimulated patterns of differentiated socialization (Maccoby 1998). If men and women are best seen to be members (and products) of distinct subcultures, then the challenge may not be to forge androgynous ideals so much as to revise or reconstruct gender-specific mental health norms.

The wide-ranging controversies surrounding gender today, outlined earlier in this chapter, complicate even this already difficult matter of embracing traditionally gendered or androgynous mental health norms. Moreover, as one of the present authors has stressed in previous writing, the very questions asked here concerning the relation of gender to norms of mental health will only receive full and thorough answers when there is open, explicit, and public discussion of the underlying values implicated (Sadler 2005). Until we have identified a vision of eudaimonia, the Aristotelian notion of flourishing, or holistic well-being—a goal not undertaken in the present work—any effort to establish how gender intersects with psychopathology must be incomplete. These ultimate value questions about how we should live, while surprisingly close to the surface in nosological debate, remain largely undiscussed, hidden from view by a medicalizing approach that emphasizes technical problems and solutions and rests on a simplified interpretation of the good life in terms of the short-term relief of individual's suffering (Sadler 2005: 238–241).

The practitioner can hardly be required to take a stand on these various questions relating to gender. Until these deeper, connected questions about the nature of the good life have received attention in a public, open discussion, the relation of gender to norms of mental health must remain uncertain, and the considerable differences and disagreements noted above, unresolved. Nonetheless, the practitioner may be required to take gender into account in several very fundamental ways and to make it a subject of therapeutic focus. If the ethical practitioner has embraced a particular position, then she will recognize and even acknowledge to the patient the status of her stance vis-à-vis its degree of certainty, as well as the fundamental values on which it rests. If she does not adopt a particular position, then she will be able to acknowledge her agnosticism over these questions.

The fact that psychiatric practice is undertaken within a masculinist setting, which puts it at special risk of reinforcing unjust and damaging power differentials, is an aspect of gender and psychiatric practice that has received considerable attention, as we have noted. That special opportunities for unethical behavior are permitted by features of the practice of psychiatry—the privacy surrounding therapeutic sessions, the intensely personal and emotional nature of the relationship, and of the material dealt with in therapy, for example—has been recognized as well, giving rise to codes of conduct governing every aspect of the therapeutic exchange. The particular vulnerability of female patients treated by male practitioners, although it still results in a disproportionate number of cases of exploitation and unethical conduct, has also been widely acknowledged (Gabbard 1989; Gantrell 1994; Quadrio 2001).

Conclusion

In light of real advances in the recognition of the gender-related problems associated with practicing psychiatry within our society, the response of the ethical practitioner must be to scrupulously abide by ethical codes. More than this, it will be argued in the chapter following this one, gender-sensitive virtues are to be found in the character of the ethical practitioner, traits that derive from the claims about gender, and the account of gender-sensitive responses outlined here. And these should be fostered.

5 Some Virtues for Psychiatrists

Introduction

Most generally, psychiatrists are professionals, so, as we saw earlier, this immediately places particular ethical constraints and expectations on them. The professional character is honorable, just, and respectful of the basic contractual relationship between provider and recipient of professional services. Virtues such as trustworthiness, fidelity, honesty, and integrity are appealed to in the very definition of professionalism, and any deviation from these traits is derogated as "unprofessional." As well as being professionals, psychiatrists are healers, and special health care virtues prescribed for those working in medical settings have been said to include benevolence, truthfulness, respect, friendliness, and justice (Drane 1988), as well as compassion, *phronesis*, fortitude, temperance, integrity, and self-effacement (Pellegrino and Thomasma 1993) and empathy (Larson 2008). Virtues judged to be especially important for caregivers within the mental health setting have included several of those above—trustworthiness, in particular—but also respect for confidentiality (Dyer 1999); compassion and humility (Christianson 1994); warmth and sensitivity (Beauchamp 1999); perseverance (Dickenson and Fulford 2000); *phronesis* (Bloch and Pargiter 1999; Crowden 2003; Fraser 2000); and caring (Bloch and Green 2006).

A comprehensive enumeration of all of the virtues possessed by the ethical psychiatrist is not provided in the discussion that follows. Instead, we focus on a collection of key practitioners' virtues, each identified through particular features of the psychiatry setting outlined previously. The main purpose of the list of virtues described here is illustrative, and that in several dimensions. Whatever way they are construed, virtues are not natural kinds. So the class of virtues is heterogeneous. This heterogeneity affects how one can proceed: the means of identifying and of habituating virtues, for example, depend on the particular virtue or virtues in question, as we have seen in the case of the empathy and personal warmth seemingly so valuable for the practitioner. The traits and clusters of traits we discuss here, then, are selected to illustrate and highlight two things: different kinds of virtues on the one hand and, on the other, different ways in which the psychiatry setting seems to call for extra virtue, and extra virtues, in its practitioners.

Virtues differ from one another in a number of significant respects. First, there are everyday and ordinary virtues or character strengths, possessed by everyone in some measure, of which the practice setting seems to call for a greater degree than do many other (including most everyday) settings. Examples of such virtues are trustworthiness, patience and persistence, self-control, and the practical good sense known as *phronesis*. On a different axis, we find traits that in everyday and other settings are ranked as useful, or as merely *prudential* virtues, rather than moral virtues, yet assume the status of role-constituted moral virtues within the practice setting. Of the virtues discussed in this chapter, realism, persistence, and propriety are virtues of this kind. Again, these are to be distinguished from the role-constituted virtue here named "unselfing," which comprises the capabilities required for proper listening and responding while maintaining the boundaries of a therapeutic relationship; in ordinary life this combination would less often be either useful or valued. Three overarching or metavirtues are also distinguishable from the clusters of traits identified thus far. One of these, *phronesis*, is the Aristotelian virtue required to size up and appropriately respond to practical situations: without *phronesis*, other virtues would fail to connect with the contingent particularities of actual experience. Another kind of overarching or metavirtue, quite different from *phronesis*, concerns itself not with the outside world of praxis but with the self or character and its unity. Examples of this type of self-unifying virtue introduced here include self-knowledge, self-unity, and integrity. The third kind of metavirtue, which we term authenticity, concerns the way in which other virtues manifest themselves. Finally some nontraditional virtues may be said to be "unruly" in requiring cultivation and habituation that is indirect, rather than direct, as we saw earlier. This kind of role-constituted virtue is illustrated by two traits: empathy, which we show to be a precondition for the virtue of compassion, and the genuine personal warmth introduced Chapter 3.

Before turning to these particular traits, we must emphasize again that virtue language is often vague, and virtues themselves inexactly and rather elastically understood. In consequence of this, several terms are employed in the following pages with little acknowledgment of the nuances that may distinguish them. Patience and persistence apparently differ little, for example, and although it has additional connotations, fortitude, too, is closely allied with those two. (Patience and persistence seem to be some of the preconditions of fortitude, for example.) In addition, each of the virtues named here comprise collections of subcapabilities, and those subcapabilities are themselves often common to otherwise different virtues. (Sensitivity and self-control, for instance, are each ingredients of a wide range of virtues.) Focusing too closely on selecting a particular virtue term will sometimes be a fruitless exercise. In that spirit, we have provided several allied terms for each of the general clusters of traits we discuss. Moreover, emboldened by Aristotle's remark that because many virtues have no names, we have to invent names for them, we have introduced one entirely new name "unselfing," to capture the attitude toward the patient required in the therapeutic setting, and we have assigned new categories, such as "gender-sensitive virtues."[1]

The virtues introduced here are loosely sorted into ten categories, without any particular ordering or any attempt at prioritization. (1) Not only as professionals, and as doctors, but as human beings, and members of society, practitioners in psychiatry will of course need to cultivate trustworthiness. We begin with trustworthiness, and demonstrate reasons why the psychiatric setting calls for extra trustworthiness on the part of its practitioners. (2) Because of the role imposed on psychiatrists through societal mechanisms of involuntary seclusion and treatment, we explore the claim, introduced in Chapter 3, that as well as being virtuous, the ethical psychiatrist will possess the virtue of propriety, taking care to avoid even the appearance

---

[1] Aristotle's passage is found at *Nichomachean Ethics* Book 2, Chapter 7, 1108a16–19, and it has been pointed out that the "nameless" virtues are all concerned with ways one should present oneself in relation to other people. (See Gottlieb 1994.)

of wrongfulness. (3) Acknowledging the importance of gender to psychiatric theory and practice, we return to the conclusions drawn in Chapter 4 about the responses of a gender-sensitive practitioner, and consider the virtues and dispositions grounding such responses. These include respectfulness, tolerance, humility, self-knowledge, imagination, trustworthiness, scrupulosity, self-control, and finally, a group of subcapabilities we entitle gender awareness. (4) The category of role-constituted virtues introduced in Chapter 3 includes traits that, while they may not be as valued, or as valued morally in other settings, are either *called for by aspects of the setting* or are *useful to healing practice*, or both. Empathy is illustrative here, since it seems to be called for by the vulnerabilities of the patient and it also plays a role in healing; we draw attention to recent work on the importance of empathy in all healing practice and to its related virtue of compassion. (The extent to which empathy is valued beyond such particular settings—and whether it ought to be valued more broadly—are issues beyond the immediate scope of our discussion, as we have said. But see, for example, Blum (1980), Slote (2004) for a fuller discussion of these matters.) (5) Like empathy in being unruly, is genuine personal warmth: this is the attribute empirical studies have shown to be a key ingredient of effective healing relationships. (6) A group of related traits focused on the self and its wholeness and coherence include self-knowledge, emotional intelligence, self-unity, and integrity. As well as the moral dangers of compartmentalization against which these self-focused virtues are directed, we note their usefulness in the healing process. (7) Certain aspects of psychiatric disorders—the uncertainties and unknowns associated with their nature and course and the controversy still surrounding them, together with the way they can compromise capabilities central to the patient's communicative and reasoning capabilities, suggest additional virtues. These features of mental illness are reasons practitioners will need to exhibit hopeful patience, fortitude, and persistence out of the ordinary. (8) Role-constituted virtues also include some that are virtues within the role morality for a particular professional practice *solely* because of their perceived usefulness. The examples discussed here are "unselfing" and realism. (9) Acknowledgment of the moral seriousness of the healing project in psychiatry seems to call for an attitude of respectfulness in the practitioner and we show the way that respectfulness will be directed toward not only the task, and the patient, but the practitioner himself, as professional self-respect. (10) Returning to earlier discussions about the demands imposed on the character of practitioners by managed care medicine, we emphasize two sorts of virtues, those required for leadership, and those for moral integrity. (11) We focus on qualities that modify the way in which almost all other virtues manifest themselves, examining the ingredients of authenticity, sincerity, or wholeheartedness. Finally, (12) because of the part played by *phronesis* in any practice and any practical endeavor, we introduce it to explore where, within psychiatric practice, its particular value might lie.

Trustworthiness or Fidelity to Trust

Trust, it is widely acknowledged, is fundamental to any professional relationship: a client needs to trust; a practitioner (whether lawyer, doctor, teacher, or any other) needs to be trustworthy. This attribute is also identified in different terms, as reliability, integrity, fidelity, or "fidelity to trust" (Pellegrino and Thomasma 1993: 135).[2] Moreover, it is arguable that rather than being a distinct virtue, such trustworthiness in the character of the professional is the precondition, or ground, for other traits accorded the status of separate virtues. (When our accountant demonstrates confidentiality, we know we can trust her with our secrets; an honest lawyer is one whose word is to be trusted, and so on.) Nonetheless, the importance of trust and trustworthiness—the social necessity of extending appropriate trust to others, and the moral necessity of being a person entitled to the trust of others—are emblematic of our lives in community, and will not here be reduced to other virtues.

These issues have received considerable scholarly attention, especially since the influential work of Annette Baier (1985, 1992, and 1995). More recently too, a virtue theory of trustworthiness has been developed by Potter, and we adopt some aspects of her account in the following discussion (Potter 2002). Potter emphasizes that being trustworthy is a matter of particular trust relations between persons, and she offers a definition of trusting relations whereby a person who is trusted and trustworthy is one who "can be counted on, as a matter of the sort of person he or she is, to take care of those things that others entrust to ... [him or her] and ... whose ways of caring are neither excessive nor deficient" (Potter 2002: 16).

---

[2] For an explication of the relationship between fidelity and trust, see Green and Bloch (2001), and for a thoroughgoing attempt to separate trustworthiness from other virtues, see Potter (2002).

Trustworthiness is not merely a professional's virtue, of course. It is a virtue probably all possess to some degree and one that, as humans and as social beings, we should all cultivate. A complex of sorts of trust structures our moral relationship with our fellows, as Baier puts it; some people must be trusted with extraordinary coercive and public decision-making powers, but *all* must be trusted as parties to promises; and *most* "trusted by some who love them and by one or more willing to become co-parents with them … trusted by dependent children, dependent elderly relatives, [and] sick friends" (Baier 1985: 60). Within this ether of everyday trust relations, our particular focus is on the *extra*, uncommon trustworthiness required of the practitioner in psychiatry, which may exceed what is usual in these several forms of trust relationship.

Potter also reminds us of some aspects of trusting relationships that explain why additional trustworthiness might be especially called for in psychiatric practice: power imbalances are a primary generator of distrust, and other problems in trust. Given the exponential vulnerability involved in trusting someone who is in a position of power over one, as she puts it, distrust "allows an already vulnerable person to be on guard against the possibility of further exploitation" (Potter 2002: 18). Where there are such imbalances, trust may be more dangerous for the one who trusts, and trustworthiness more important in the one placed in a position of trust.

The power imbalances which Potter notes are often systemic and structural based on how institutions and social relations are organized; to greater and lesser degrees, they will affect everyone's trust. More immediately applicable to us are the imbalances between practitioner and patient resulting from the patient's several vulnerabilities. Such imbalances are a function of many things, not all of which are systemic: societal attitudes, but also the characteristic symptoms and uncertain course of much severe mental disorder, the isolation and neediness of its sufferer and, in the treatment setting, the importance of confidentiality. There, as in the everyday settings of which Potter writes, trust and power intersect, and those with more privilege or power—here, practitioners—"have proportionately more work to do to give assurances which *indicate* a trustworthy character" (Potter 2002: 17, our emphasis).

Trustworthiness will be a virtue of special importance to the practitioner in psychiatry, then, at least in part because the inherent power imbalance in the therapeutic relationship, and the relative powerlessness of the patient, powerlessness likely to have engendered distrust. The practitioner can build trust in two ways: by cultivating a degree of trustworthiness which overcomes such distrust and, as the emphases we have imposed on Potter's passage makes clear, by making extra efforts at *demonstrating* her trustworthiness to the patient. The practitioner must be able to be trusted and also show she is to be trusted.

Further considerations suggest why the virtue of trustworthiness will have special importance for the practitioner in psychiatry. That practitioner, we saw, is "entrusted" with the special and morally weighty public safety responsibility of committing and treating the dangerous mentally ill against their wishes. Practitioners are trusted to be judicious, careful, and fair in all their dealings but particularly here, where their role affords them such a great power over other, innocent adults. Again here, it should be noted, the practitioner will need to *be* a person of extra trustworthiness but may also need to demonstrate that trustworthiness to distrustful others. The psychiatrist has special duties incumbent in this societal role, we shall argue presently, and must possess virtues allowing her to undertake this communicative effort of *showing or demonstrating her moral character*, including her trustworthiness.

Finally, trustworthiness is a useful—perhaps the most useful—virtue for any medical professional, widely believed to be required for any effective treatment. Trusting one's practitioner may not itself promote healing, but trust in one's practitioner seems almost certainly a condition without which other agents of healing could not take place. Recognition of this has been part of medical lore since Hippocratic times, and it was well understood, for example, by the great Persian philosopher and physician Avicenna. Adding his own commentary to this long recognized medical understanding, Robert Burton reminds us that "because the Patient puts his confidence in him, which Avicenna prefers before art, precepts, and all remedies whatsoever … And he doth the best cures, according to Hippocrates, in whom most trust" (Robert Burton 1948: 223).

Trustworthiness then is a quality essential to practice. And because the ease with which trust can be engendered in others is sensitive to power imbalances, and the psychiatry setting is replete with such imbalances, the practitioner is called on to possess, and show, greater trustworthiness in this than in many other settings. The corresponding temptation or character weakness here will be that of failing to achieve, but also failing to demonstrate and convey, this heightened trustworthiness.

Public Appearances and the Virtue of Humble Propriety

Charged with the power of civil commitment, the psychiatrist must meet not only the ethical demands of the immediate situation but the additional demand of conveying public appearances consistent with virtue. (See Chapter 3.) This imposes a substantively higher moral standard on the practitioner than on other professionals or on ordinary citizens. But the moral significance and weight of the public and political role society has assigned to practitioners demands, and justifies, such a standard.

There are close parallels between the demand that practitioners in psychiatry exhibit such propriety and appearance standards sometimes applied to public officials. To maintain public trust government servants are required to act so as to avoid fostering a reasonable belief that they have been guilty of any wrongdoing in the mind of the public. And like elected officials, we argued in Chapter 3, psychiatrists act as society's representatives in undertaking the public safety role assigned to them. Members of the community must be able to trust them, and that trust is essential for the maintenance of these important societal institutions ensuring public safety. Required to override the autonomy of citizens neither guilty nor even suspected of any crimes, psychiatrists must not only do the right thing but also uphold the public trust imposed on them by avoiding the appearance of wrongdoing.

Arguably, the person who maintains the public appearance of virtue is simply one whose character is exceptionally virtuous by dint of possessing greater integrity, more trustworthiness, deeper compassion, and so on, and who goes to extra lengths to demonstrate the presence of each of those traits. On that view, conveying the appearance of virtue will reduce to conveying the appearance of whatever other virtues the person possesses. In our analysis, by contrast, publicly appearing virtuous will be conceptualized as its own separate and distinct virtue.

The trait or traits involved in appearing virtuous are here named "propriety," since the concept of propriety most aptly captures these habits of carefulness over appearances. We want to emphasize that propriety is an important virtue and not merely a superficial or even hypocritical *show* of proper behavior. The virtue of propriety comprises a distinct set of motives, as well as many different, internalized patterns of attention, care, and sensitivity to the effects on others of one's behavior and words; in addition to communicative skills and understanding, they also include strengths of forbearance, self-control, and self-knowledge. To effectively convey the appearance of a person possessed of a virtuous character is its own moral challenge; to do so habitually requires sustained moral effort.

The virtue of propriety is one called for by the psychiatry setting, rather than useful for healing practice. Arguably, indeed, this virtue is one that might at times prove inimical to a strong therapeutic alliance.[3] (When the practitioner is perceived to be a paragon of virtue, for example, the patient may suffer by the comparison with herself.) The qualification above, that links this virtue to public appearances, may assuage some of these concerns: such propriety may not be called for in the relative privacy of the therapeutic setting, where virtue alone may be sufficient, without its outward show. Nonetheless, to the extent that this tension remains, the practitioner whose societal role requires propriety while her obligation to healing directs her to foster the therapeutic alliance is burdened with something close to conflicting roles. Role conflicts are not infrequent for practitioners in psychiatry, we will see in the chapter following this one, because of the several additional societal goals practitioners are called on to uphold, not only public safety, but criminal justice and national security. We do not mean to diminish the genuine moral dilemmas and tensions that arise this way. But we note that the potential for misunderstanding associated with a demonstration of the appearance of virtue (the danger of appearing superhumanly perfect, arrogant, or "holier than thou") are part of the exacting demands of the virtue of propriety. Propriety, as we define it here, must also embody a stance of suitable humility, effectively conveyed.

Being virtuous will always be more morally important than appearing to be, needless to say. And in comparison with many other virtues, humble propriety will perhaps always remain a minor virtue, even in the psychiatry setting. Nonetheless, the moral importance and great societal power entrusted to the psychiatrist require that she cultivate and demonstrate propriety, which will enable her to maintain the public appearance of a virtuous character. The character weaknesses and temptations corresponding to propriety include, most immediately, carelessness over appearances. But, because the practitioner's narcissistic inclinations will likely be fed by this morally elevated appearance, additional vices can be expected to involve a failure of self-awareness of humility or both.

---

[3] We are grateful to several practitioners for drawing our attention to this tension.

Gender-Sensitive Virtues

We saw in the previous chapter that several aspects of our culture and the practice of psychiatry come together to make gender issues inescapable ethical concerns to which the practitioner must respond with seriousness and imagination. Gender cannot be ignored, nor the healing project be undertaken without attention to the patient's own presuppositions about gender and gender identity. The broad historical context is one in which the nonmale, nonmasculine, and homosexual have been disfavored and often pathologized; the contemporary culture is still masculinist in many of its structures and *de facto* functioning; gender categories are central to the identity at the heart of the healing practice of much psychiatry; and enormous controversy surrounds gender issues. Such realities, we saw, necessitate a certain character in, and particular responses from, the ethical psychiatrist. Here, we review these responses and see what would most effectively ensure them through the cultivation of entrenched dispositions in the practitioner.

One of these responses concerns the patient's gender identity. When severe mental disorder is present, basic cognitive and communicative capabilities may not permit the patient to determine his own gender identity. When those capabilities remain unaffected, we saw, the ethical practitioner has reason to allow the patient to not only assign his own gender from the spectrum of possibilities, but also, perhaps, to evaluate that gender assignment and identity—as healthy or unhealthy, acceptable or shameful. Ceding the authority to the patient in this way, we would again emphasize, has analogies in changes that have occurred in other areas of medical practice as the result of new thinking in biomedical ethics. The principle of informed consent, for example, has largely replaced earlier paternalistic models in which the best interests of patients were dictated by the medical team and regarded as part of the practitioner's specialized knowledge. Explaining the ethical reason for giving authority to the patient when decisions about her best interests are involved, theorists have appealed to the principle of autonomy and the respect owed persons by dint of their humanity. Patient autonomy has become one of the most—and arguably the most—widely honored principles within biomedical ethics (Beauchamp and Childress 2001; Bloch and Chodoff 1981; Bloch, Chodoff, and Green 1999; Edwards 1997). The disposition identified and honored when we understand this principle in *aretaic* terms is respectfulness of that autonomy.

Such respectfulness for the patient's autonomy may also apply to ceding authority to the patient over gender assignment and identity. (This would be to find a place for the "recognition rights," noted earlier, which have been the focus of identity politics.) In these circumstances, we suggest, the ethical practitioner will be called upon to respond with empathic understanding and imagination. She will likely encounter ideas, ideals, and gender identities unlike her own. To respect her patient, she will need to place herself, imaginatively, in her patient's place, and see the world through his eyes. This kind of empathic understanding is not easy and not without its dangers, as recent work on empathy has shown (Halpern 2001). Empathy, which allows the practitioner to imagine how it feels to experience something, for example, cannot be confused with either detached insight, or affective merging. (We return to the notion of empathy later in this chapter.)

The controversy surrounding gender concepts today combine with the presumption from identity politics that a nondelusional person should be accorded the privilege of self-definition when it comes to gender identity to discourage an ethical practitioner from offering assessments about the patient's gender. The ethical practitioner will grant her knowledge that may be incomplete or, if she has embraced a particular account of gender, will be prepared to acknowledge the theoretical and perhaps ideological status of her opinion. These attitudes, we saw, are likely to embody two traits, tolerance (of other practices and norms and other forms of gender identity) and the humility born of recognition that the practitioner's own ideas and attitudes about gender may contain misapprehensions, parochial prejudices, and unwarranted assumptions.

In a discussion of the character requirements for any psychiatric practice, Leston Havens has singled out the virtue of modesty. This is an attitude, he explains, appropriate in light of any particular practitioner's incomplete understanding and single, limited perspective (Havens 1987: 95). Undoubtedly, Havens is right in emphasizing that such modesty or humility will always be appropriate. But it will be all the more so, we would stress, when the practitioner's perspective concerns matters as controversial—and as linked to self-defined characterization identity—as gender. To the virtue of respectfulness of the patient's autonomy, then, must be added these virtues of tolerance and humility.

Further virtues may be called for here as well. The ethical practitioner need not, and perhaps should not, adopt a particular account of gender.

(Given the uncertainties surrounding gender outlined in Chapter 4, even the adoption of a provisional theory of gender may detract from the open-minded tolerance and humility apparently required in the practice setting.) But she will need to make gender a subject of discussion. This suggests that the ethical practitioner will have some understanding of her own gender ideas, ideals and identity, in order to guard against inappropriately imposing them in such an exchange. As an individual situated within a gendered practice in a gender conscious society, such self-knowledge will be an essential trait and, given its centrality to practice, a role-constituted virtue.

Added to these virtues of the gender-sensitive practitioner are the traits required to avoid the sexual exploitation of patients. As we have seen, psychiatry is practiced within a broader cultural setting that puts it at special risk of reinforcing unjust and damaging power differentials already magnified by the vulnerability of many in the patient group involved; this invites particular emphasis on trustworthiness in the practitioner. Only hard-earned trustworthiness demonstrably entrenched in the psychiatrist's character will be a remedy against the opportunities for unethical and sexually exploitative behavior that are part of psychiatric practice.

In response to such opportunities and temptations arising in the practice of psychiatry, it is true, carefully considered rules, prohibitions and guidelines have been codified for practitioners. And by scrupulously adhering to such codes, the ethical practitioner can avoid the temptations inherent in the practice setting. But scrupulosity and self-control, while important, are not the only virtues required here. Since self-interest alone might dictate obedience to such rules, the presence of appropriate motivation will be important as well. The ethical practitioner who is gender sensitive will be aware of the reasons behind these rules; she will appreciate not only the practical and professional consequences but the moral significance of abiding by them. And these reasons will function as motives for her. The virtue underlying this extra appreciation of such codes of conduct, we suggest, can simply be called gender awareness.

The temptations and character weaknesses against which gender-sensitive virtues are a remedy have sometimes been thought so magnified by the situation in which male, heterosexual practitioners treat female heterosexual patients that the virtues required of those practitioners would need to be different from the virtues required of other practitioners. Our view, in contrast, is that the diversity of gender identities, together with the controversy increasingly surrounding traditional binary distinctions about gender, will require that all practitioners adopt and foster all gender-sensitive virtues.

To recapitulate: the several virtues required for gender-sensitive practice, we can now see, will mark the character of the practitioner with the traits of respectfulness, tolerance, humility, self-knowledge, imagination, trustworthiness, scrupulosity, self-control, and, finally, gender awareness. The character weaknesses and temptations against which these virtues should prove a remedy include not only those involving the sexual exploitation of patients but the tendency to accept conventional wisdom and ideological lore as scientific fact; failures of imagination; and a want of those intellectual virtues we associate with an open mind.

Empathy (and Compassion)

The notion of role-constituted virtues was introduced in Chapter 3, where we saw that two distinct rationales seem to be identifiable when we consider the character of the psychiatrist. Many virtues are called for in practitioners simply because of the particular practice setting. The vulnerabilities and suffering of the patient, the profound significance of the therapeutic project, the roles assigned to the psychiatrist by society—these all introduce ethical expectations that can be understood as demands for a certain kind of moral character in the practitioner. And these virtues are called for regardless of any usefulness they may have for healing practice. The compassion prompted by another person's suffering and vulnerability, for example, is an expression of our common humanity and requires no further explanation or justification in terms of social role.

Some of these role-constituted virtues, by contrast, ought to be cultivated because of their usefulness to practice—their apparent link with therapeutic effectiveness. The trait or traits making up empathy provide an important example here for several reasons. First, psychology increasingly grounds feelings of compassion in the primitive, probably unlearned and mimetic tendency to empathize (Brothers 1989; Gallese 2003; Halpern 2001; Hoffman 1984, 2000; Hurley and Chater 2005; Ickes 1997; Levenson and Ruef 1992; Larson and Yao 2005; Prinz 2005).[4] Although that tendency is apparently

---

[4] As Prinz has sketched it, for example, infants and young children have a tendency to imitate others that allows them to feel and respond to what others feel and so acquire what he calls "moral comprehension" (Prinz 2005: 267). Thus "if an infant recognizes someone's distress by 'catching' it, the infant will in effect be distressed by that person's distress" (Prinz 2005: 275).

natural, education is required to ensure the "empathic arousal" (Hoffman) that is found in morally responsive adults (Hoffman 2000). Eric Larson and Xin Lao have recently emphasized the "emotional work" of empathy-building in medical education (Larson and Lao 2005). They speak of this labor as the process of "regulating and displaying emotions to present a professionally desired image during interpersonal transactions" (2005: 1103). If we understand empathy as a precondition for the general virtue of compassion described above, then empathy can be understood as an aspect of compassion rather than as a separate trait. But empathy has also been identified as a state or capability *useful* for those engaged in healing practices. Thus two, distinct considerations mark empathy as a key role-constituted virtue in the practice setting. It is necessary both because of its link to the compassionate responses called for by that setting, and because of the part it plays in healing.

Empathy is an everyday virtue, present to some degree in everyone and, like trust, an essential ingredient of moral and social life. In the following discussion, then, it must be noted, "empathy" refers to a *degree* of empathy greater than that found in all, or at least all morally responsive, adults.

The therapeutic effectiveness of empathy has not always been recognized. At one time, empathy referred to the tendency toward "projection" (attributing one's inner states on another person) or even, borrowing from a long association with aesthetics—where empathy is a merging between the feelings of the observer and the artist—by imagining the others' experiences to be one's own.[5] In his 1957 essay on the necessary and sufficient conditions of therapeutic personality change, Rogers introduces something closer to our present day notion of empathy, as a heightened interpersonal sensitivity and understanding *free of projection or merging*.[6] For healing to occur, Rogers insists, the therapist must experience an empathic understanding of the client's internal frame of reference and must succeed in communicating to the client that this understanding has been achieved. Such empathy was not in order to better know about the patient's frame of reference, however. It was to convey the experience of being understood. For in that experience, Rogers believed, lay the source of healing (Rogers 1957).

In more recent work, introduced earlier, Halpern employs a model of empathy that shares much with Rogers's concept and that, although it does not explain empathy in *aretaic* terms, can be readily adapted to cast the

---

[5] The term "empathy" is from the Greek *empatheia* for "feeling into."

[6] Similar recognition of the distinction between true empathy and such merging is found in Scheler 1970.

tendency or capacity to respond with empathy as a character trait (Halpern 2001). Halpern defines the person possessing empathy as one who, by using her imagination, can "resonate emotionally with, yet stay aware of, what is distinct about the patient's experience." This account of empathy utilizes the idea of participating in another's experience, but rejects the model of merging in favor of one in which the imaginative use of the practitioner's affects thus provides a "framework, or organizing context, for understanding the patient's particular experience" (Halpern 2001: 85).[7] Halpern emphasizes the use of the imagination.[8] In recent experimental studies the "feeling with" aspect of empathy has also been tied to more perceptual capabilities: detecting another person's fleeting feelings through facial expression and other nonverbal cues, in order to identity specific cognitive states in others (Ickes 1997). We may suppose then that the subcapabilities making up empathy comprise both the imagination and more perceptual skills of noticing and other forms of recognition.[9] Clearly, these are capabilities that can be harnessed in the clinical setting to enhance healing.

---

[7] Interestingly, many of the distinctions that emerge from Halpern's analysis are to be found in earlier witing about compassion by Lawrence Blum. Blum defines compassion as a "complex emotional attitude toward another, characteristically involving imaginative dwelling on the condition of the other person, an active regard for his good, a view of him as a fellow human being, and emotional responses of a certain degree of intensity" (Blum 1980: 509). Blum emphasizes the extent to which compassion depends on the imagination and shows that imaginatively reconstructing another's condition must be distinguished from a merging identification with the other that would actually prevent true compassion (Blum 1980: 507–-517). Similar features are noted by Beauchamp and Childress's definition depicting empathy as not only an active regard for another's welfare but an imaginative awareness and emotional response of deep sympathy, tenderness, and discomfort at another's misfortune or suffering (Beauchamp and Childress 1971).

[8] John Deigh has emphasized that more mature forms of adult empathy involve an understanding of what it is to live a human life—the recognition of others, as he says, as architects and builders of their lives. Such mature empathy involves recognizing others as autonomous agents and "participating imaginatively in their separate lives" (Deigh 1995: 760). In a related distinction, Robert Gordon notes that imagining in being another person's situation is different from imagining being that other person in their situation. The empathy required to foster the therapeutic relationships and described by Halpern seems to presuppose both the maturity noted above and the complex imaginative stance portrayed by Gordon (1995).

[9] For a discussion of the subcapabilities allowing us to be affected through contagion yet also recognize the separation between our own and others' affective states, see Gordon (1995).

Empathizing with patients who are suffering is useful to healing practice in two distinct ways, Halpern argues. First, it allows the practitioner to discover more about the patient's experience, and thus treat more effectively. An additional healing effect derives from the *sense of being accompanied* experienced by a person whose situation is responded to with empathy. This is close to the mechanism Rogers envisioned.[10] The function of empathy in such cases, according to Halpern, in a kind of "burden-sharing" effect that "helps ... the sufferer to feel the full scope of intensely aversive affects, such as overwhelming grief or fear." A patient, Ms. G., is described, whose suffering has left her locked in a despairing view of her life. For Ms. G., the practitioner's empathy permits the return of a healing curiosity: she simultaneously "takes herself seriously and ... becomes curious about her convictions about the future" (Halpern 2001: 113–114).[11]

If Halpern's causal claims for the usefulness of empathy are accurate, empathy of the kind she describes should be part of the character of the ethical practitioner because of the effectiveness with which it furthers the goal and good of healing. However, empathy is doubly important for the ethical practitioner. And in ending this discussion we want to emphasize that *regardless* of the usefulness of empathy in the healing process, the state of patients like Ms. G. and the isolation, suffering, and pain endured by many patients with psychiatric conditions seem to call for the quality of empathy and the compassion of which it is a precondition and central ingredient. Their common humanity will require such responses from practitioners in the face of the palpable suffering, neediness, and vulnerability that the practice setting of psychiatry so frequently reveals.

Empathy is closely related to the personal warmth introduced earlier, as we saw. (At the very least what makes such warmth possible will be the same subliminal capabilities making empathy possible.) Like warmth, for example, empathy appears to be an unruly trait: admonishing ourselves to feel empathy will not make it happen. Imagining, noticing, listening, and reasoning to "read" others' minds, and so on are all actions we can undertake at will, however. So the habituation of the virtue of empathy that takes place where trainees are enhancing their ability to empathize within the

---

[10] Others have pointed to the healing effect of a closely allied feeling of being understood (Charland and Dick 1995: 416).

[11] Halpern also argues that empathy is the interpersonal support necessary for developing a sense of self-efficiency; such empathy is evident in parents as they develop a sense of agency and self-efficacy in their children.

training setting can be undertaken indirectly, just as can the task of engen-dering warmth. Although they may have originated in subpersonal mimetic tendencies well beyond conscious awareness or control, such capabilities may be enhanced through education and training, as Halpern's and much other research indicates.[12]

A particular feature of the psychiatry setting is the long-term and uncer-tain nature of much severe mental disorder rendering many mental patients potentially long-term patients. Luhrmann sees this aspect of psychiatry as calling for a particular kind of empathy in the practitioner. "Simple" empathy and its compassion, as she puts it "help sufferers only when the suffering can go away" it is the empathy structured by the biomedical model that separates the person from the disease. Complex empathy, in contrast, is called for by suffering that is woven into the complex web of a person's past and identity. You cannot feel for this person simply that he is a victim of a depression the way he might be a victim of the latest hurricane, for "the hurricane of depres-sion is part of who he is, and to emphasize with him is to empathize with his self-destructiveness as well as with his despair" (Luhrmann 2000: 277). Approaching these cases with simple empathy will actually be detrimental to healing and to the sufferer's dignity. "If people's personhood is independent of their psychiatric illness but the illness never goes away ... What it is to be human in them—thinking, choosing, feeling—is sick, and is out of their con-trol" (Luhrmann 2000: 278).

Luhrmann may be right that there are two separate forms of empathy. But as we saw in earlier discussion of identity and illness, this relation is depicted in different and sometimes incompatible ways by those enduring or having experienced mental disorder. The nature of the symptoms (their severity and quality, for example); the patient's understanding of self and identity, and degree of adherence to the tenets and assumptions of biologi-cal psychiatry, will all influence these matters and affect the plausibility of Luhrmann's claims. We are at least in broad agreement with Luhrmann that the potentially long-term aspect of psychiatric disorder has implications for the self-identity of its sufferers that will in turn affect the degree, if not the kind, of empathy called for.

For practitioners, the character weaknesses or temptations correspond-ing to empathy and compassion will be all those tendencies inclining them

---

[12] The Self Science curriculum used in primary education includes much effective empathy training, for example, Stone and Dillehunt (1973). But see, also Rest (1986), Goleman (1995), Deigh (1995).

away from caring about their patients: failures of attention, imagination, and heart. Some of these will be due to moral weaknesses, such as narcissistic self-regard. Others, of course, will result from less culpable stresses and strains incumbent in practice. The unfailingly empathetic and compassionate practitioner is, after all, an idealized one.

Warmth (and Genuine Warmth)

The role-constituted virtues of personal warmth, together with genuineness, are attributes consistently identified as effective in the therapeutic relationship, we saw. Yet both seem to be loose concepts, not easily captured in a precise definition. Warmth involves congeniality, agreeableness, and a readiness to like and respond positively to others. As a practitioner's virtue, it cannot solely be a disposition to experience feeling states. It will embody a sort of understanding of the worth and personhood of the other and perhaps also of the broader professional good involved, a recognition of that warmth is what the other person needs.

Personal warmth differs in two respects from several of the other virtues we have discussed here, such as trustworthiness and patience. First, it is not valued in all contexts: it is admired by some people less than by others, in some cultures more than others, and its appropriateness and acceptability are often judged relative to context and social role. Perhaps it ought to be more widely valued than it is. But, arguably, it has little or no place in many everyday and professional settings, where mere competence and skill, or stern neutrality, seem to be preferred traits. Second, as we saw earlier, it is unruly, apparently springing from traits that are so internal or internalized as to be described as "natural," or "innate," and inaccessible to attention, reason, and direct self-control. This unruly nature, we believe, is compatible with regarding personal warmth as a role-constituted virtue. In contrast, genuineness is not a virtue, as such. Rather, it is a quality attributable to any character trait (as in a "genuinely funny" man, or a "genuinely caring" one). To attribute genuineness to a person *tout court* seems to be to say little more than that she genuinely possesses her other virtues.

The way in which warmth is genuine differs from the way more traditional virtues such as patience, or trustworthiness, are deemed to be genuine. If a person is genuinely patient, or trustworthy, it is because he has habituated the actions comprising that virtue in something like the way the Aristotelian model proposes and is wholehearted and sincere in his response. Because warmth is unruly, ensuring genuine warmth is a different kind of task, as we saw earlier, and genuineness is attributed differently. The well-intentioned practitioner in the therapeutic setting who has intentionally manipulated her feelings to exude warmth may be morally admirable. Yet still we might resist describing her warmth as genuine. Genuine warmth is required to be not merely heartfelt, but *unstudied*—so deeply internalized as to have become an unthinking habit.

The weaknesses and temptations corresponding to genuine warmth, then, will be several, led by personal coldness, aloofness, and indifference. False, or even studied warmth, must be included, as must warmth which is an indiscriminate emoting without real understanding of the person to whom the warmth is directed. Again, a failure to communicate or somehow convey warmth (however genuine) must count as a weakness in the treatment setting where the warmth that is called for must be perceived or recognized by the patient. As this series of failings suggests, getting it right, with genuine warmth, is a demanding goal—getting it entirely right, always, is probably an unreachable one. Nonetheless, striving toward that ideal, we believe, is what the ethical practitioner should do.

Self-Knowledge, Emotional Intelligence, Self-Unity, and Integrity

No two virtue or trait terms are exactly synonymous. But the blurring between virtues and groups of virtues makes it difficult and perhaps not finally useful to try to distinguish them too meticulously. Whether we speak of a person's character as trustworthy, or as exhibiting fidelity, for example, an explication of this trait into more particular dispositions and responses will likely reveal the same or similar subcapabilities. This sort of confusion and blurring is evident when we approach the cluster of traits associated with what is commonly known by philosophers as self-knowledge or self-understanding, and by clinicians and social scientists as insightfulness or self-awareness.

Characterized as understanding one's own subjectivity, psychic states, and traits, including one's character, self-knowledge is bound to other qualities in at least three distinct ways, and we introduce and discuss them in turn here. First, understanding oneself is allied to understanding other persons. The broad trait of emotional intelligence studied in psychology, for instance, comprises skills that allow for both intrapsychic and interpsychic knowing. And because of their role in understanding and empathizing with others, these traits are relied on in the practice setting of psychiatry. Second, although self-knowledge does not always ensure a unified self, it is closely linked to self-unity, and we explore below the relationship between the traits of self-knowledge and self-unity and their apparent contribution to effective practice. Finally, self-knowledge has widely been understood in philosophical traditions to stand as a precondition for the transparently moral virtue of integrity and associated self-regarding and wholeness-regarding qualities often judged necessary for any virtuous character. After commenting on each of these separate aspects of self-knowledge, we close this discussion by pointing out the status of self-knowledge within our culture's norms of mental health.

Knowledge of Oneself and Others

Recent efforts to pull away from the cognitivist bias of past psychological trait analyses have led to an acknowledgment of a plurality of different "intelligences" including a social intelligence, found in the linked abilities to understand oneself and other people. Variations on this idea have emphasized the part played by emotions in such capabilities, providing an analysis into a number of subcapabilities, of what has come to be called emotional intelligence. One set of these subcapabilities includes perceiving and appraising emotions, assimilating emotional experiences, motivating oneself, understanding and reasoning about emotions in others, and handling relationships—that is, managing emotion in oneself and others (Mayer et al. 2000: 400; Salovey and Mayer 1990). A similar analysis more focused on achievements or "competencies," and social outcomes, includes emotional self-awareness, managing emotions, harnessing emotions productively, empathy, or reading emotions, and handling relationships (Goleman 1995: 283–284).[13] A recent discussion defines emotional intelligence as the ability to "assimilate emotion in thought, understand and reason with emotion, and regulate emotion in the self and others" (Mayer et al. 2000: 396).

Like several of the other role-constituted virtues introduced here, emotional intelligence is not a moral virtue in everyday life; it is simply recognized

[13] Because it introduces social effects, this second model has been described as a mixed, rather than a mental abilities model of emotional intelligence (Mayer et al. 2000: 403).

as an extremely useful asset (Goleman 1995; Mayer et al. 2000; Peterson and Seligman 2004).[14] And virtues are traits, not achievements. Yet clearly these contemporary notions of emotional intelligence capture many of the attributes likely to enhance practice in the psychiatric setting. For example, the subskills of emotional intelligence include, or at least seem to ensure, empathy—and empathy, as we saw earlier, is effective in healing. And strengths in "motivating oneself" (Mayer, Salovey and Caruso) and "harnessing emotions productively" (Goleman) suggests tools for employing indirect means to instill the several unruly virtues believed so essential to effective practice in psychiatry. Thus we propose that as it is understood by psychologists, emotional intelligence, together with its range of intrapsychic and interpsychic subcapabilities, is an additional role-constituted virtue.

Self-Knowledge and Self-Unity

Self-knowledge and self-unity are not easily separated. Each usually requires an exercise of reflective self-examination, for example. And they are often sought, although perhaps not always found, together.[15] We can of course envision a degree of *fragmentary* self-knowledge that is neither motivated, nor accompanied, by a unified psyche. Yet it would be but fragmentary, and an incompletely unified psyche would correspond to such partial self-knowledge. Self-knowledge and self-unity are perhaps separate qualities, conceptually, but as dispositions they are difficult to prize, and keep, apart.

Self-knowledge and self-unity, it seems very likely, are traits required for therapeutic effectiveness. To the extent that the practitioner does not know herself, and her own weaknesses and innermost preoccupations, those weaknesses and preoccupations could blind-side her in the therapeutic encounter, impeding its effectiveness. (Her own unresolved feelings about an issue raised by some detail of her patient's narrative, for example, might prevent her from attending to, or later recalling, that narrative. Nonverbal

[14] How much this quality corresponds to the practical intelligence known as *phronesis*, discussed later in this chapter, will perhaps determine the full force of this claim. As we have defined these qualities, emotional intelligence cannot be equated with *phronesis*.

[15] Alternative paths to a unified self than the self-conscious and rationalistic efforts associated with acquiring self-knowledge have been proposed by thinkers such as Martha Nussbaum and Nomy Arpaly (Arpaly 2003; Nussbaum 1996).

indications of surprise, annoyance, or indifference reflecting an insufficiently integrated psyche, would seemingly detract from the delicate relationship with her patient, and so on.)

A further reason why physicians must cultivate self-knowledge follows from their particular social position. Noted by Drane, this was introduced in Chapter 3: self-knowledge will be a remedy against the temptations and vices that come with privilege and powerful status. Physicians, as Drane puts it, "are vulnerable to self-ignorance and self-deceit because they are persons of power and privilege. People cater to them and infrequently tell them the truth about themselves. As the top authorities … doctors usually get their way … It is easier for doctors to see the faults of others than to see their own faults. As a result, it is easy for doctors to develop a narrow and conceited view of themselves, frankly to become fools when it comes to their inner truth … " (Drane 1995: 61–62).

At least two separate features of the psychiatric setting make self-knowledge and self-unity important virtues for practitioners, then: the value to the therapeutic alliance of a unified and insightful self in the practitioner, and the temptations incumbent in the practitioners' status as medical authorities.

Self-Knowledge and Integrity

The notion of integrity is etymologically akin to "integration," and the relation of its part to a whole, so a person of integrity will be one who is in some way unified and coherent. The relation of self-knowledge to such wholeness is introduced here; later in the chapter, when we consider the virtues of practitioners in the particular context of managed care, we will return to look at integrity from a broader perspective.

As a central concept in moral philosophy, the notion of integrity has received notably different analyses. Reviewing some of these, Cheshire Calhoun distinguishes an "integrated self" view (the integration of one's desires, evaluations, and commitments into a whole), from an "identity" view (fidelity to the projects and principles constitutive of one's core identity). A third, "clean hands" view (where integrity involves maintaining the moral purity of one's own agency) is more explicitly normative (Calhoun 1995).[16] One way to

---

[16] Calhoun introduces her own view of integrity as "standing for something," which stresses the social context in which integrity must be understood, which is one in

differentiate these approaches to the self-integration or wholeness of the person distinguishes psychological accounts (corresponding to "self-unity" as it was introduced earlier) from more normative ones that place formal, evaluative limits on the kind of person who might be said to possess integrity.

While distinguishable, these psychological and moral analyses are closely connected, however. Just as self-unity is often sought through self-knowledge, so the coherence and consistency of integrity understood in normative terms seems often to depend on a quality of psychological coherence and consistency. An integrated psychological subjectivity apparently augers, and may even be a precondition for, integrity understood in moral and not merely psychological terms.[17]

Moral integrity is commonly believed to be called for by the fundamental relationship between all professionals and their clients. It is such integrity, as May puts it, which "makes possible the fiduciary bond between the professional and the client," signifying as it does "wholeness or completeness of character" (May 1994: 87). If any professional practice depends on moral integrity in the practitioner, so it in turn depends on self-unity in the psychological ("integrated self") sense, and so on self-knowledge. (This is not to say that coherence and self-unity are the sole ingredients for moral integrity or that moral integrity can be reduced to the possession of these self-unifying traits.)

Within the role morality adopted here, it must be remembered, no distinction can be maintained between what are customarily thought of as moral, or character, virtues (such as moral integrity) and useful traits (such as self-knowledge and self-unity). For the practitioner in psychiatry, self-knowledge and psychological self-unity are also moral virtues, even if "self-unity" is not defined in explicitly normative terms.

Self-Knowledge and Self-Unity as Mental Health Norms

It may also be true of other role-constituted virtues introduced here, but it is particularly true of the traits of self-knowledge and self-unity that they comprise some of the norms of mental health that shape practice. Whatever other

which a person stands up for his/her own judgments in a community of "deliberators" seeking moral value.

[17] For this reason, attempts to avoid traditional conceptions of the self while putting forward a theory of integrity seems doomed to be unsuccessful (Cox et al. 2003).

personal changes patients seek, their aspirations will almost inevitably entail self-knowledge, and often some form of self-unity, as well. The patient's is a normative project: improvement or betterment of some aspect of her own life and self is sought. As such, the traits, dispositions and habits of mind making up self-knowledge and self-unity will enter that project, either as ends in themselves, or because of their perceived instrumentality in bringing other goals, such as enhanced well-being, or autonomy. Though often incompletely or imperfectly achieved, such goals underlie even the most fleeting and superficial encounters in psychiatry. The patient seeks to understand herself more fully and often to gain a more unified and coherent self as well. Similarly, a striving for a more ambitious and moral kind of integrity has also been attributed to patients and to the psychotherapeutic project (Glover 2003; Lomas 1999).[18]

We attribute these goals to psychiatric patients with some confidence in part because as a normative project, psychiatry will always be culturally embedded, reflecting the prevailing values and ideals of the broader social context in which it is practiced. And that context, we want to emphasize, attributes value—at least to the extent that they do not jeopardize richness and variety of personality—to self-knowledge and self-unity. Such cultural embeddedness has more commonly been recognized in relation to other ideals, such as autonomy and effective social and occupational functioning. Particularly with the decline in psychoanalytic and psychodynamic psychiatry during the last decades of the twentieth century, these latter values of autonomy and effective functioning have received more explicit recognition than the ideals of self-knowledge and self-unity. Nonetheless, we believe that the normative project in psychiatry continues to be influenced by the cultural and personal ideals that derive from two legacies—that of the unitary and integrated self of Western individualism, on the one hand, and insightful and introspective modern self, on the other. As A.C. Tjeltveit has pointed out, these values are deeply ingrained in our culture, preceding, and likely to far outlive, the particular influence of psychoanalysis: "Ridding ourselves of pleasant self delusions, courageous self-scrutiny, and an honest view of ourselves were ideals shared by Nietzsche and Freud" (Tjeltveit 1999: 160). Ineluctably, as mental health norms, self-unity and self-knowledge help to shape more particular therapeutic goals.

---

[18] See Lomas, for example: "an assessment of whether the patient's moral stance is a true expression of his being is central to any therapeutic undertaking" (Lomas 1999: 57).

Tjeltveit indicates the sort of character weaknesses corresponding to the role-constituted virtues of self-knowledge, emotional intelligence, and self-unity outlined here. Ignorance of one's own inner states due to "pleasant self-delusions;" cowardly failures of self-scrutiny and a dishonest view of oneself are the first—these will prove hindrances to therapeutic effectiveness and healing. And so too will failures to understand and know others' inner states arising from inattention, insensitivity, and forgetfulness. A tendency toward the disintegrated self that MacIntyre names "compartmentalization," which is the particular character weakness corresponding to self-unity or integrity, will be explored more fully later in this chapter.

(Hopeful) Patience, Fortitude, and Perseverance

The group of character strengths variously described as patience, fortitude, and perseverance are common virtues, recognized within everyday spheres as well as role-specific ones. They are widely agreed-upon as valuable, and widely deemed necessary for every imaginable setting. Their central ingredient is an ability to persist with a plan or task even in the face of difficulties, to "stay the course." Because they are primarily behavioral in their make-up, to *exhibit* patience, fortitude, and perseverance is almost to *have* these traits. Thus they may be successfully feigned. (Seething with annoyance inside, one may still be able to exert enough self-control to appear patient.) Additional subcapabilities of such traits, then, include self-control and an ability to conceal what may be incompatible or inappropriate inner states.

When genuine, these virtues include an ability to maintain an unwavering confidence in the worth of the task or plan of action, a kind of hopefulness. And this trait, in turn, will convey hope and engender it in the patient—an element of considerable value to healing, as recent survivor memoirs, and discussions of recovery, repeatedly make clear (Bracken and Thomas 2005; Davidson 2003). A key ingredient in psychiatric rehabilitation, hope has been described as "the belief that no matter how severe the illness, how chaotic the life, how depleted the resources, there is always the possibility of small steps of recovery" (Wakeman 2002: 118).

The value of hopefulness as a character trait in the practitioner is one that has been recognized for some time. (See Havens 1987; Mann 1997.) And in a more complete account of the character of the virtuous psychiatrist it would receive fuller treatment, we acknowledge. Here, however, it is introduced as an ingredient in patience, fortitude, and perseverance as a spirit in which such attitudes are adopted and maintained.

Many of the difficulties, frustrations, and challenges faced by practitioners in the psychiatry setting that demand their patience, fortitude, and perseverance, pertain to the nature of the therapeutic project and of mental health care. Others derive from the sometimes conflicting roles and responsibilities imposed on the practitioner, who must on occasion compromise the trust and healing components of the alliance in order to comply with, for example, public safety obligations. (One of these obligations is the legal [Tarasoff] duty to warn, after a patient has expressed intent to harm others.) When there is such conflict of roles, the sense of having violated the patient's trust will be a painful and irksome one, calling for the resolve and strength of fortitude.

So many social roles and life circumstances demand these virtues that it would be an exaggeration to claim that the psychiatry setting is one in which they are more required than in any other. Nonetheless, we want to point out features of the psychiatry setting that make these traits essential, and likely call on more patience, hopefulness, fortitude, and perseverance, in the character of the practitioner than do some other medical settings, at least. Four such features, introduced in Chapter 2, provide particular reasons why the virtuous psychiatrist will need these traits in abundance. First, as we said earlier, severe mental disorder frequently affects interpersonal responses, including reasoning, attitudes, moods, and communicative capabilities. At least from time to time, this will require the practitioner to struggle during communicative exchanges in order to follow reasoning, appreciate attitudes and affective states and, in some cases, merely to understand what is being conveyed. That such communicative problems arise in other medical settings is undeniable. (The comatose patient cannot communicate at all, for example.) But to the frequency with which communicative capabilities are compromised this way in the psychiatry setting, must be added another distinctive feature of that setting. There is an unusual reliance on such communication with the patient when treating disorders that are without the *independent forms of verification* so common in other areas of medicine (scans and tests, for example). These factors combine to magnify problems of communication in psychiatry. So, in turn, they serve to augment the demands on the practitioner's capacity for patience, fortitude, and perseverance.

The unusually complex and ambivalent attitudes psychiatric patients often have toward their symptoms, noted in Chapter 2, constitute a second aspect of the psychiatry setting calling for these traits in the practitioner. Examples of such attitudes, as we saw, include the pleasing energy of mania, or the grandiosity of paranoia, making these desirable conditions. Unaccompanied by the customary attitudes and expectations associated with more ordinary medical symptoms—acknowledgement that such symptoms indicate disorder, and a desire to cooperate in their removal, for example—psychiatric symptoms often interfere with a communicative exchange involving the set of understandings and expectations around what Talcott Parsons called the "sick role" (Parsons 1951). Considerable perseverance is required in the practitioner, who, before the healing project can continue, must undertake, and frequently reiterate, basic interpretations concerning those expectations.

A third reason for extra virtue of this kind in the practitioner stems from the fact, also noted earlier, that some unidentifiable cohort of patients will prove to be long-term patients, suffering a recurrence of disorder. Taking this long view, the practitioner must treat every patient and every exchange with complete attention and perseverance. There can be no place here, for example, for the impatience to be finished we associate with many tasks nearing completion. Such a feeling is one of the vices against which the virtues of patience, fortitude, and perseverance are a remedy. A second such vice is losing heart in the project. The long-term aspect of many cases of mental disorder, and uncertainties as to their course, also call for an unwavering hopefulness in the practitioner.

Finally, the controversy surrounding mental disorder will likely put extra pressure on the character of the practitioner. Every aspect of professional practice, theory, and lore of psychiatry is in our society subject to questioning and skepticism, and this is true to a much greater degree than is true for other branches of medicine. In the face of such challenges, and of quite widespread misunderstanding from the community, to maintain unwavering confidence in the value of the healing task, and hopefulness over particular outcomes must require comparably greater effort from the practitioner. To endure, when one's professional role is so frequently challenged, will take a degree of dogged staunchness, even "fortitude."

Each of the features of the psychiatry setting we have noted here will magnify the need for the everyday virtue of patience, perseverance, hopefulness, and fortitude. Other roles and life circumstances may demand even greater quantities of such virtue than the psychiatry setting. But among other medical specialties, psychiatry seems to be unusual, at least, if not unique, in the need for this group of character strengths in its practitioners.

The temptations and character weaknesses that correspond to this cluster of virtues, the above analysis seems to suggest, include all forms of impatience and frustration over disappointing progress: a wish to be done and to move on; a tendency to boredom when the way is tedious; losing heart in the project; despair, discouragement, and pessimism.

Unselfing and Realism

Some role-constituted virtues are relatively practice-specific. We here focus on two of these, "unselfing," defined below, and realism. Though not moral virtues on traditional definitions (on the Aristotelian schema, unselfing is not a virtue at all, and realism is at best a prudential virtue), each of these are professional's virtues inasmuch as they are useful or even necessary for effective psychiatric practice.

The term "unselfing" here refers to the personally effaced yet acutely attentive and affectively attuned attitude toward the patient, the relationship, and its boundaries, adopted by the ethical and effective practitioner.[19]

This trait has some parallels in the attitudes required of all professionals toward their clients. Any recipient of an expert's paid services is entitled to that professional's undivided attention; moreover, "boundaries" are established and maintained, with greater and lesser degrees of care, around most professional relationships. (Conflicts of interest are regularly codified and proscribed, for example.) In part because of the extra vulnerability of many psychiatric patients, and in part because of the belief that more casual or everyday elements in the relationship will likely interfere with the effectiveness of the alliance, concern over maintaining the formal "frame" around the psychiatric relationship is unprecedented, however. The concept of unethical boundary infringements or "violations" has given rise to an elaborate codification of every nuance of gesture, conduct, and communication in the therapeutic relationship, to a set of metaphors, and to the vocabulary (of boundaries, the frame, boundary crossings, and violations), which is the *lingua franca* of much informal psychiatric ethics discussion today.

[19] Pellegrino and Thomasma draw attention to the need for what they call self-effacement, but self-effacement here is placed in contrast the self-interested and narcissistic attitudes these authors attribute to an overweening self-centered individualism in modern culture; it is not the same as unselfing as we are introducing the notion here (Pellegrino and Thomasma 1993:144).

The broad rationale for maintaining this heightened attention to boundaries, introduced earlier, has considerable acceptance. Such boundaries, as we saw, have been represented as a constraining structure within which the usual psychological boundaries respected in interpersonal exchange can, between patient and therapist, be crossed with safety (Gabbard 1999: 143). Maintaining the personally effaced yet attentive attitudes toward the patient that make up what we are entitling unselfing is generally agreed to be central to the ethical and effective psychiatrist's professional role, although how it is employed will vary with the kind of therapeutic engagement.

Unselfing plays a different part in the character of the ethical psychiatrist from that of self-knowledge and self-unity. Although not moral virtues outside of the setting in which they constitute virtues for practitioners, self-knowledge and self-unity are widely valued as intellectual virtues; indeed, they are even emblematic of mental health. Unselfing, in contrast, seems to have little currency in everyday life. In ordinary relationships, the attentiveness, sensitivity, and care associated with being a good listener is valued, it is true, and unselfing includes those traits. But in everyday settings, at least in our culture, we also value mutuality, and an equality of exchange. Indeed, like emotional detachment, reserve is sometimes judged a hindrance to intimacy and mutuality, and thus, *prima facie*, unappealing. (If such reserve were judged wrongful, then the practitioner's adoption of the virtue of unselfing might seem to indicate an instance of the less defensible, strong role morality that requires responses considered to be unethical within broad based morality. But greater emotional openness and a tendency toward more mutual and conventional exchanges would seem in everyday, broad based morality to be prudential virtues at best, not moral ones.)

Unselfing must be distinguished from the attitudes of detachment required of all professionals, which have been the subject of considerable philosophical attention and analysis (Appelbaum 1991; Appelbaum and Jorgenson 1997; Curzer 1993; de Raeve 1996; Oakley and Cocking 2001; Fried 1976; Halpern 2001; Postema 1980). As a professional, the psychiatrist may also need to adopt an attitude of detachment in response to some of the demands of the psychiatry setting. And such detachment undoubtedly bears some similarity to unselfing. Like unselfing, for example, detachment requires vigilant self-control. But the differences here are telling.

First, in contrast to unselfing, professional detachment involves an emotional distancing from the states or plight of the client: a Stoic denial of one's own feelings in favor of a controlled, unemotional "professionalism." The practitioner in psychiatry monitors her feelings and their expression, it is true, but she does not expunge them. Indeed, she must experience and often communicate aspects of inner states—of warmth, empathy, compassion, and acceptance, for example. Her feelings are an essential part of the healing effort. Second, unselfing imposes much broader limits on self-disclosure than those regulating professional detachment—not only her reactions and responses, but factors about her social and cultural background, ideas, and many other facets of nonprofessional life.[20] Third, while professional detachment is controversial, the elements making up unselfing represent a readily justified divergence from more mutual relationships. The "alliance" between practitioner and patient is so important and so dependent on the practitioner's attention to boundaries that maintaining and supporting the relationship through the exercise of the role-constituted virtue of unselfing is a critical ingredient in therapeutic success. Unselfing is essential to healing.

Several of the character weaknesses and even vices corresponding to unselfing are well known: exploiting the patient, in whatever fashion, violates the boundaries of the relationship. But to those must now be added sheer carelessness over boundaries, including various forms of unwarranted self-disclosure, and insufficiencies of emotional engagement, such as inattention and insensitivity.

Realism is not always a trait valued in everyday life, although it is more valued in some settings than others; but when honored, it is customarily as a prudential virtue rather than a moral one, important in promoting one's own good. Realism implies that one's thoughts, beliefs, and responses are kept in line with the facts, as the facts are understood by those around us.[21] The realist maintains a balanced view, moreover, steadily adhering to the perspective and evaluations suggested by those facts. In this respect realism includes the kind of equable and consistent view of things that others have described as perspective (Tiberius 2002). In everyday life realism is a trait so commonly encountered in adults that it is somewhat humdrum, and lapses

[20] As we noted earlier, there remains considerable disagreement, based in part on theoretical differences, over how far these limits on self disclosure extend.

[21] The realism which is a virtue for practitioners is not to be confused with the metaphysical realism that makes claims as to the nature of truth: realism in the sense under discussion here concerns the intersubjective agreement, or reliability, of beliefs.

from it—common, and all too human—and even from this rarer trait of perspective, are generally attributed to carelessness or self-deception.

In the treatment setting, however, realism is an important virtue. Here, it is called for owing both to characteristic symptoms of mental disorder itself and to the nature of the healing project. If only temporarily, severe mental disorder often deprives patients of the capabilities contributing to the trait of realism. Severe symptoms of delusion and hallucination have even been characterized as a failure to distinguish reality from a subjective and delusional unreality. Kant long ago pointed out an important feature of much mental disorder, indeed for him the "only general characteristic" of insanity: "the loss of a sense of ideas that are common to all (*sensus communis*), and its replacement with a sense of ideas peculiar to ourselves (*sensus privatus*)" (Kant 1978: 117). With the severely disordered patient, interpretations by the practitioner often convey the *sensus communis* against which the *sensus privatus* can be judged. For the psychiatrist, then, the humdrum prudential virtue of realism will become a moral virtue in the treatment setting.[22]

Some forms of therapy explicitly presuppose that the practitioner corrects mistaken beliefs and evaluations in the patient: in such cognitive-behavioral modes realism in the practitioner is a cornerstone of healing (Erwin 1978, 2004). The practitioner will likely be required to demonstrate and exemplify realism for the patient in many other forms of treatment as well, however. (It should again be emphasized that the practitioner is not an arbiter in the sense of identifying what is real, so much as identifying and modeling the "facts" as they correspond to intersubjective and public agreement.) Humdrum as it is, realism also represents a prudential virtue in our culture

---

[22] The psychiatric project invites some comparison with the somewhat analogous—and certainly analogously profound—task of fostering a child's emotional and intellectual growth and forming its character, carefully explored and described by Sara Ruddick. Among the virtues demanded by this morally significant and culturally essential task Ruddick notes several nontraditional traits including realism. A young child must learn realism as it comes to know and interpret its world, and because realism is a deeply relational trait, in which appeal is made to the thoughts, beliefs, and responses of those around us, this requires a nurturer equipped with the trait of realism to act as teacher and guide (Ruddick 1995: 98–101). The analogies here are not exact, but Ruddick's emphasis on the relational nature of this trait serves to explain why the practitioner, just as the nurturing parent, must foster the role-constituted virtue of realism.

and thus a mental health norm, we must add. As such it will likely be sought in the normative project undertaken by almost all patients.

The character weaknesses and temptations corresponding to the role-constituted virtue of realism would include tendencies toward any interpretation of the facts diverging from intersubjective realities, whether the product of idiosyncrasy, ignorance, arrogance, or willful blindness to those realities. In particular, realism would seem a strong preventive against the overvaluation and self-centeredness of narcissism, and the self-deception and want of self-doubt that, we saw, may be engendered by medical status.

Respect for the Patient and the Healing Project

Respect for other persons and, in particular, for the person of the client is an important, widely-acknowledged virtue for all practitioners in all professional roles. Solely as a professional, the virtuous psychiatrist will possess this attitude of respect for the personhood of every patient encountered in the clinical setting.

The worth of persons for which an attitude of respect is so widely deemed appropriate has been understood philosophically in two rather separate ways. One tradition represents it as ours merely by dint of being human. That worth is said to be unearned, invariable, and inalienable. Differently understood, attitudes of respect for persons are linked more closely to conceptions of merit. Earned, variable, and alienable, it is a kind of worth that may vary from person to person. Separating these two conceptions into "dignity" and "merit," respectively, Robin Dillon explains that "The grounds for *dignity* are variously said to include a person's intrinsic nature (as a person, an autonomous agent, a moral agent), or such things as one's status in a rigid social hierarchy, cultural heritage, or identity-conferring membership in a particular class or group. The grounds for *merit* include an individual's character and conduct insofar as it reveals character; as well as those traits, qualities, abilities, and accomplishments that are important from a moral point of view or from the point of view of the individual's living out her plan of life" (Dillon 1995: 21, our emphasis).[23]

For the professional, we may conclude that very often both grounds will contribute to, and warrant, an attitude of respect for persons toward the

---

[23] Interestingly, the notion of desert also spans these two distinct conceptions: people are said to "deserve" respect for both reasons.

client (or patient). Such respect will be owed because the client or patient deserves it, as a human being, a person, a moral agent. It will also be adopted in recognition of her "character and conduct"—those traits, qualities, abilities, and accomplishments that are important from a moral point of view. Applied to the patient in the psychiatry setting, such traits, qualities, abilities, and accomplishments have been noted earlier in this book. They include, for example, the courage, persistence, ingenuity, and frequent effectiveness shown by those who live with debilitating psychiatric symptoms, and the virtues of the "good patient," noted earlier: not only persistence and courage, but honesty, hopefulness, flexibility, and trustfulness, for example.

The moral significance of the healing project in psychiatry, where, as we saw, disorder affects the cognitive, affective, communicative, and volitional attributes closely associated with personhood, also calls for an attitude of respect. (See Chapter 2.) Such a profound task, we want to emphasize, demands a practitioner cognizant of its moral seriousness. Insufficient, and even morally inappropriate here will be the stance of a mere technician toward the possession of a skill. Recognition of the moral significance of the trust imposed, given the nature and moral gravity of the project, seem to ask for something akin to a respectfulness that extends beyond the patient to the task itself.

Such an attitude is perhaps closest to what Paul Woodruff describes as the ancient, and almost forgotten, virtue of *reverence* (Woodruff 2001). Woodruff defines reverence as "a sense that there is something larger than a human being, accompanied by capacities for awe, respect, and shame" (Woodruff 2001: 63). Of the vice corresponding to this particular virtue, he remarks, "Ancient Greeks thought that tyranny was the height of irreverence, and they gave the famous name of hubris to the crimes of the tyrants. An irreverent soul is unable to feel awe in the face of things higher than itself" (Woodruff 2001: 4). These definitions suggest the theological antecedents of the concept. But reverence may also be the appropriate attitude toward something that is merely larger and more morally weighty; more valuable than at first appears, or than it might customarily be taken to be. (Great art, for instance, or great human goodness, both invite the attitude of reverence. Although neither is, in Woodruff's words "larger than a human being" in any theological sense, each is beyond ordinary human capability.)

Even setting aside the theological connotations of reverence, the explicitly evaluative language and presuppositions introduced here may be resisted, for they are antithetical to much in modern day psychiatric lore. Just as Freud was, most practitioners today seem reluctant to acknowledge the moral significance of their task (Rieff 1959). This reluctance may stem from a biological conception of medical science that strives to avoid moral concepts and categories. It may also derive from a modesty—misplaced, we believe— which leaves practitioners unwilling to exceed what they regard as their field of skill and expertise. Reflecting as it does the influence of the consumer model wherein the practitioner has been assigned the role of purveyor of technical services, however, this very language (of skill and expertise), we hope to have shown, is insufficient.

Some observers have acknowledged the additional, normative aspects of the practice of psychiatry, it is true, although there is not agreement over the extent to which psychiatric practice today already is, or ought to become, a moral enterprise. Speaking of such practice, Peter Lomas asserts that "we are in the realm of the moral rather than that of science, and we stand or fall by our practical wisdom rather than our technique" (Lomas 1999: 103). Similarly, Luhrmann, whom we quoted earlier, observes that psychiatry is inevitably tangled with "our deepest moral concerns: what makes a person human, what it means to suffer, what it means to be a good and caring person" (Luhrmann 2000: 23). The focus of Luhrmann's work was the incompatible worldview and philosophical presuppositions dividing the psychodynamic perspective from the biological one, incompatibilities leaving practitioners conflicted and ambivalent. But her exploration of the culture of late twen- tieth century psychiatry sees validity in both views, and finds both views embraced by practitioners. Despite their ambivalence and conflict, despite the discomfort they may feel in such a moral role, Luhrmann found that practitioners often recognize the broader, moral aspects of the enterprise in which they are engaged.

The virtue of respect for the healing project, we suggest, may be charac- terized somewhat differently. We have proposed that it involves respect for the person of the patient, in both senses identified above, and that it involves an attitude of something close to reverence for the moral seriousness of the project itself. These attitudes, we surmise, will in turn generate a degree of self-respect or faith in oneself on the part of the practitioner. Although as Woodruff pointed out, irreverence can lead to hubris, there is a kind of pride in oneself that is virtuous, and it is this pride, or self-respect, that seems to complete the attitude we are attempting to characterize here. The practitioner who possesses the virtue of respectfulness toward the healing task respects the person of the patient, acknowledges and honors the moral seriousness of the undertaking and, in addition, respects herself for undertaking it.

The role-constituted character weaknesses and temptations that corre-spond to the virtue identified here imply three kinds. First, there is a failure to respect the patient, both as a person *simpliciter* and as one who struggles often valiantly against many odds. A second aspect of the related character weakness is a kind of misplaced scientism that prevents recognition of the moral seriousness of the therapeutic project. And finally, there is a kind of misplaced modesty—a devaluing of one's own work and role that will likely lead to a denigration of one's efforts and retreat into the role of purveyor of technical services.

Virtues for Managed Care Medicine: Moral Leadership and Moral Integrity

The managed care setting within which psychiatry is increasingly practiced, we saw in Chapter 3, presents its own challenges and has been seen to call for certain character virtues in practitioners more vital today than they were in earlier practice regimes. Here, we focus on two of the several virtues which managed care psychiatry seems to demand, moral leadership, and moral integrity.[24]

Earlier, we introduced Chervenak and McCullough's emphasis on the moral leadership required of doctors in managed care settings. Today individual phy-sicians discharge their fiduciary obligations in and through institutions, these authors explain, requiring them to take on responsibility for the "moral culture of health care organizations." It is morally incumbent on physician-leaders to ensure that medical responsibilities, values, and goals, such as the fiduciary professionalism of physicians with daily responsibility for patient care, medical education, and research, are reflected in the organizations within which they practice. Only management skills and the cultivation of a new set of moral virtues will equip physicians for moral, medical leadership.

The particular virtues advocated by these authors are self-effacement, by which they mean impartiality in the face of differences of status, class, gender, and race; self-sacrifice; compassion; and integrity. These traits must

---

[24] Loretta Kopelman has provided a useful discussion about the moral traits required for managed care medicine, but her focus is not on particular virtues (Kopelman 1999). Kopelman enlists Humean moral theory to explain how the partiality demanded of doctor–patient relationships can be reconciled with, and is even a precondition for, the impartiality required for just health care systems.

be fostered and their corresponding vices (of unwarranted bias, inappropriate self-interest, hard-heartedness, and corruption, respectively), eschewed.[25] The physician-leader who consistently uses institutional power and authority to advocate for these professional virtues of the physician as a moral fiduciary, they observe, together with physician–patient relationships that are based on these virtues, will " crucially support physicians as the moral fiduciaries of their patients" (Chervenak and McCullough 2001: 878).

That same virtue of moral leadership prompted by the advent of managed care systems has directed some theorists to consider additional values beyond protecting fiduciary roles (Minogue 2000; Povar et al. 2004; Sabin 1994, 1995). Now other, broader aspects of these delivery systems, including "stewardship" and resource use, have been recognized as part of the new portfolio handed to today's medical leaders. The central challenge for creating ethical managed care systems, James Sabin has insisted, is not merely protecting fiduciary values but integrating stewardship responsibilities to the whole society with the patient centered values practitioners have always tried to uphold (Sabin 1995: 293).

Integrity is a second virtue whose importance has been emphasized by those concerned over the bureaucratic structures that come with managed care. Alasdair MacIntyre's plea for integrity arises in a discussion of the dangers of compartmentalization engendered by any large, impersonal bureaucratic organization (MacIntyre 1999). Such organizations encourage a separation and segregation of roles, each governed by its own specific norms in relative independence of other such spheres. To ward off the moral dangers this decentralized structuring invites, MacIntyre proposes the cultivation of the virtues of integrity (sometimes also referred to as constancy).

MacIntyre's first and most telling example is the German functionary, a man who perfects his duties in making the trains run, wholly failing to question whether their cargo may be Jewish deportees instead of pig iron. Looking back on this kind of dedication to the duties of a role, MacIntyre insists, we do ask more of the functionary than fulfilling his duty as a small part in a larger system. We hold him responsible for not looking beyond his closely defined role.

---

[25] These virtues, Chervenak and McCullough note, derive from two eighteenth-century English thinkers, doctors John Gregory (1724–1773) and Thomas Percival (1740–1803) whose ideas, in their view, define "the professional nature of the doctor–patient relationship to this day (Chervenak and McCullough 2001: c876).

MacIntyre's reasoning appears to rest on several key ideas. To be full moral agents (as the German functionary was not), we must understand ourselves, present ourselves to others, and possess a sense of ourselves as independent of the sum of the roles we play and we need to see ourselves as rational inquirers, entitled to and confident in our judgments. To question and evaluate the institutionalized system in which we are a part we must adopt a role-independent stance.

An "integrated self" analysis of integrity is employed here, focused on psychological and moral wholeness, and the self recognized as a role-independent identity. MacIntyre believes these traits are engendered and maintained through dialogue with others. Only such dialogue will ensure the critical and evaluative stance afforded role-independent identities. MacIntyre's definition of such integrity was quoted earlier: "to refuse to be, to have educated oneself so that one is no longer able to be, one kind of person in one social context, while quite another in other contexts...to have set inflexible limits to one's adaptability to the roles that one may be called upon to play" (MacIntyre 1984: 317).

MacIntyre depicts integrity as a trait manifested by standing aside from one's various role responsibilities in order to evaluate the system from which those responsibilities have arisen. The ability to avoid compartmentalization by standing apart from one's roles, and questioning and evaluating the system or systems from which they emanate, is an achievement, MacIntyre emphasizes, and not easily attained. But with help from others it can be: "this ability requires participation in social relationships and in types of activity in which one's reflective judgments emerge from systematic dialogue with others and are subject to critical scrutiny by others" (MacIntyre 1999: 321).

If MacIntyre's thesis is defensible, then it seems to offer valuable suggestions about managed care ethics. For ethical practice in managed care settings it will be necessary to possess not only those virtues such as compassion and benevolence with direct bearing on practice situations, but also the moral integrity associated with role-independent identities. As a central ingredient in the cultivation and maintenance of these role-independent identities, consultation with others will be required. The maxim customarily employed in clinical practice hitherto has been "when in doubt, seek consultation." But MacIntyre's insights indicate the insufficiency of such a rule. Consultation is not valuable merely as a way of clarifying hard cases and dilemmas, and avoiding particular moral pitfalls such as boundary violations. In addition it is at the heart of being a full moral agent.

In reflecting on the character weaknesses and temptations against which the virtuous practitioner must guard in the managed care setting then (at least as these two analyses showed them), we must include failures of moral leadership, together with compartmentalization, and finally, an unpreparedness to engage in dialogue and consultation with colleagues.

Authenticity, Sincerity, and Wholeheartedness

The quality known as genuineness, as we saw earlier, is complex and even ambiguous. When attached to personal warmth, it requires not only an unfeigned and sincere effort, but a natural or unstudied one. For virtues more straightforwardly habituated than warmth, however, the assessment that they are genuine implies only that they are sincerely and wholeheartedly felt and conveyed. It is this latter, simpler sense of genuineness, also captured by terms such as "authenticity," "wholeheartedness," and "sincerity" that is intended here. It is an attribute that attaches to a way of possessing other virtues, and thus what might be termed another kind of metavirtue. And it is one of particular importance because of the temptations that permit and even invite the practitioner to feign virtues. Feigning can be defined as exhibiting, with the intention to deceive, the manifestations associated with some inner state (a feeling, disposition, belief, motive, or attitude), in the absence of that inner state. None of the nouns we have employed to capture the positive attributes making up the virtue we are concerned with here ("authenticity," "sincerity," "wholeheartedness") is without confusing additional connotations of its own. Yet because the opposite of this trait is familiar and easily recognized, little further needs be said as to its characteristics. It is the same attribute that Rogers names "congruence" and defined as a match between a person's inner feelings and outer display (Rogers 1957). (For Rogers it was the first of three conditions necessary and sufficient for healing, we add.)

Feigning and deceit occur everywhere, it is true.[26] But in everyday contexts people can frequently recognize insincerity and pretense, discerning real from feigned responses and "reading" one another's inner states and character. These cues, we believe, are often not afforded the patient in the psychiatry setting.[27] Aspects of that setting that might prevent the

---

[26] The moral and policy implications of this are not inconsiderable (Gehring 2003).

[27] Interestingly, Kittay argues that the particular wrongfulness of hypocrisy is that it stands in the way of this reading of inner states from outward actions and

patient from knowing the practitioner well include the rigorous "boundaries" placed on the psychiatric engagement. Although appropriate and necessary, these restrictions serve to limit the patient's capacity for discerning which responses are genuine and which feigned. A second aspect of the setting is that, although falseness and hypocrisy show themselves most readily when *actions* belie words, the practitioner's actions are often limited, and the contrast between deed and word so revealing of falseness, is rarely available to the patient. Also interfering with the patient's ability to identify feigned responses will be the delusions, projections, and other communicative problems of social awareness and response associated with some symptoms. The combination of these features will make successful feigning easier in the mental health care setting than in many others, a fact confirmed by history: from antiquity until the modern era, "pious frauds" and deceptions to trick patients were an accepted mainstay of treatment for various mental disorders (Jackson 1999).

That said, the heterogeneity and variability of virtues will limit the degree to which they may be feigned in a range of ways. Since they cannot be effected at will, forced efforts to display expressions of unruly virtues seem likely to be ineffectual. In contrast, virtues more closely associated with particular motivation than with particular feelings, it would seem, will be easier to feign. Showing a pretended respectfulness for the patient and the healing project, might be an example. Granted, successful feigning of respectfulness will also call for a degree of sensitivity to the context and setting, and that sensitivity may not be so easy to contrive. But if that sensitivity is present, as a learned trait or a natural talent, then pretended respectfulness may be possible also. Virtues also vary in the extent to which they are tied to their inward or to their outward manifestations. Courage, to use one of Aristotle's examples, reduces to, or at least is very strongly associated with, its outward manifestations in the form of courageous actions. This is confirmed by the way we speak. To "*show* courage," as we say, is to be courageous. (The courageous man may even *feel* frightened, indeed according to Aristotle, he should feel [the right amount of] fear.) Showing courage may not be easy. But, if what is required is the appropriate outward response, it will likely be easier to feign courage than some other virtues. Of the virtues explored earlier in this chapter, we saw that patience had this characteristic as well. (And notice

expression. As she says "The hypocrite severs the act from the intention...[and] undermines our belief in the appearance as being anything other than appearance" (Kittay 1982: 285).

that here, too, we speak of a person's "*showing* patience.") An outward show of patience can successfully conceal inner states of impatience. In yet another modality, variations occur in the extent different virtues are characterized by discrete and easily recognizable sets of outward manifestations. The virtue of patience, for example, comprises a combination of characteristic inner and outer manifestations, but as we just saw, because of the distinctiveness of its outer manifestations, it may be successfully affected. Harder to feign will be sensitivity, the shape of whose outward manifestations eludes any characterization in terms of a finite set of appearances, gestures or actions. The perception, attention, and understanding required for possessing the trait of sensitivity are inner states that determine the outer form it will take: the actions, demeanor, and response called for.

Feigning may not be as egregious a vice as many others, and in a later chapter (Chapter 6) we demonstrate that, as an aspect of the habituation model of virtue cultivation, less culpable forms of feigning will be, for the learner, inescapable. Nonetheless, as the vice against which the virtues of authenticity and wholeheartedness are remedies, it is a danger, we believe. There is a kind of misplaced modesty that encourages today's clinicians to see themselves as mere technical experts, as we saw earlier (Radden 2008). Since some of the traits we have identified as role-constituted virtues are importantly instrumental in therapeutic effectiveness, the practitioner in psychiatry may be tempted to see her personality or *persona* as a healing instrument analogous to a surgeon's scalpel and thus to conclude that skillfully feigned traits would be as effective as unfeigned ones—the appearance of honesty, pretended sympathy, a superficial display of trustworthiness, and so on. A skillful practitioner would then be thought to act ethically in feigning, and perhaps even be required to feign, these qualities. Again, we want to insist, this is a temptation which practitioners ought to resist, and against which they will need to instill the virtue of authenticity.

The Metavirtue of Phronesis

In Aristotelian theory the virtue of *phronesis* (usually translated as practical wisdom or as intelligence) stands as the humbler, practical analogue to the more intellectual, theoretical *sophia* (wisdom). Both are broad capabilities. *Sophia* enables us to study and know the truths of science and philosophy, while *phronesis* allows us to deliberate about things with ends or goals in mind, and to discern and enact right action. A grasp of particulars is required for *phronesis*, so it comprises cleverness (in the ability to find what is needed to achieve an end or goal), perception (in order to notice facts in a situation), and finally, understanding (*noûs*), a common and practical good sense. *Phronesis* is a kind of metavirtue for Aristotle, guiding action in every situation and implicated in the appropriate manifestation of all other virtues. When right action occurs, it is as the result—and demonstration—of *phronesis*.

Several contemporary thinkers have found an important place for the virtue of *phronesis* in healing practice (Bloch and Pargiter 1999; Crowden 2003; Fraser 2000; Kronman 1987; Megone 2006; Pellegrino and Thomasma 1993). Recognition of this particular fit comes from the way medical practice concerns, and *phronesis* is the virtue to deal with, matters that are uncodifiably particular, and not reducible to orderly principles.

The difficulty of making the case that *phronesis* has special applicability here, whether in psychiatric practice or in medical practice more generally, is that *phronesis* is useful everywhere in practical life. Its importance is at least assured in any professional setting where a provider of services interacts with a client, be it dentistry, accountancy, or law. So while acknowledging that this virtue will be needed in psychiatry, a little more must be said to explain its distinctive applicability to this setting.

Pointing to the need for *phronesis,* Fraser has noted that both diagnosis and treatment in psychiatry require an application of theoretical knowledge to particulars. In diagnosis, using reflection, or deliberation, "the psychiatrist must move beyond analysis, separation and labeling…to an understanding of the particular person in his individual context" (Fraser 2000: 3). Treatment, similarly, involves deliberation: "The appropriate use of medication is essential to the effective treatment of psychiatric disorders. Knowing when and how to utilize psychological interventions is equally vital to effective treatment. The psychiatrist needs the right academic knowledge of these treatments, and also the perceptiveness to discern the needs of the patient" (03–04).[28]

---

[28] Our discussion of the place of virtues in psychiatric practice has thus far focused on practitioners as clinicians, yet many clinicians are also researchers and research itself calls for special virtues in those engaged in it. The research setting is not the focus of this book, and the moral character of the researcher will not be explored here. But one important discussion of the virtue of integrity has taken this challenge seriously, and it must be acknowledged. Pellegrino and Thomasma point out that the virtues of the scientist are those that enable the scientist to attain truth: they list such virtues as objectivity, critical thinking, honesty in recording

Similar to Fraser's recognition that the effective practitioner will require *phronesis* is Brendel's stress on the importance of adopting a pragmatic approach to psychiatric practice. Mental disorders are complex, Brendel explains, and "treating them usually occurs in the face of significant uncertainty." When there is sound empirical evidence for the efficacy of a treatment, "clinical ethics demands that the evidence be heeded. But in cases where there is less certainty (or no relevant empirical evidence at all), clinical decision making should not be wedded to any particular theory at the expense of concrete, practical considerations" (Brendel 2006: 39–40). *Phronesis* will surely be called for in decisions such as the pragmatic ones Brendel describes and if, as he suggests, psychiatric practice is unusually complex and uncertain, then arguably the demand for *phronesis* will be greater in this than in other settings.

Paying attention to the particularities of every circumstance, as it does, *phronesis* is not one among equals with other virtues. Rather, it is a kind of metavirtue, in the sense of determining which other virtues will be applicable given those particularities. In what might almost be seen as an adjudicative role, it must then be involved with the relationship between the other virtues. Imagine a scene in a therapy session: the patient struggles to

and reporting data, freedom from bias, and sharing of knowledge with the scientific community (Pellegrino and Thomasma 1993: 135). In addition, however, they point out that society places trust in scientists, so they add trustworthiness, or what they call the virtue of fidelity to trust. "The public provides funds, facilities, and the conditions conducive to free inquiry in the expectation that they will be used to expand human knowledge for the benefit of all. Those who accept funds for research enter into a covenant with society in which the primary goods cannot be power, personal profit, prestige, or pride" (135). These authors go on to point to the temptations for researchers in what they call the "industrial model" of research where, as they put it, research is a commodity like any other, an item produced for its exchange value, for what it yields in promotion, tenure, lighter teaching loads, a larger laboratory, more support dollars, and so on.(page 136) "the scientist must cope with a series of challenges inherent in the complex fiscal, professional, and social structure of contemporary scientific research. These challenges all conduce to the vice of selfish self-interest. At every turn, there are inducements to self-interest that subvert the purposes of research and violate the public trust. P 135 Such an inducement is provided by pharmaceutical companies, they point out. They conclude that "the ubiquity, urgency, and complexity of these changes in the structure of research that follow its industrialization are serious threats to the integrity of the investigator...[making it] even more compelling morally to do whatever we can to prevent scientific misconduct" (Pellegrino and Thomasma 1993: 137).

speak, fighting back sobs. Is this the moment for a gesture of sympathy and affirmation—or for immobile, attentive listening? The practitioner possesses both sympathy and patience, but which virtue should find expression in this particular, emotionally charged moment? Resolving that practical quandary will require *phronesis*, the virtue that consists in being able to see what matters and what is to be done.

The distinct tensions between some of the attributes of the virtuous psychiatrist identified in previous discussion suggest a further reason why there may be a special place for *phronesis* in psychiatric practice. (Some of the same, or similar, tensions may arise in other medical practice, but we want to concentrate on those apparently heightened by the demands of the psychiatry.) Several examples of these tensions have been introduced already, of which we will focus on two. The first involves the carefulness over appearances named in this book propriety. Such a virtue, we saw, might at times conflict with the need to convey acceptance and a nonjudgmental attitude in a therapeutic setting: patients would likely be intimidated, or moved to invidious comparison, in the face of such an appearance of perfection in the therapist. The therapist must avoid appearing "holier than thou" then, adopting appropriate humility; at the same time, though, he must eschew even the appearance of wrongfulness in all public conduct. Here is a situation and tension in response to which only experience, sensitivity, and a remarkable degree of *phronesis* will be equal, we suggest.

A second example involves the rigorous demands of the disposition here named unselfing in a situation where, as we saw, genuine personal warmth was also called for. How can the clinician maintain such strict monitoring of her every word, expression, body language, and gesture, to the point of great apparent personal reserve, while at the same time successfully conveying a positive regard for the patient that will be perceived to be desirably "genuine" and "natural"? To emphasize the almost paradoxical nature of these demands: *How can she not be herself, while at the same time being completely herself?* Again, the answer must lie with the presence of *phronesis*. She can do so because she possesses the ability to see what matters and *what is to be done*: how, in what way, and at which moment to reveal the warmth she feels; how, in what way, and when to demonstrate the self-effacement and reserve that are required by unselfing.

A different way in which *phronesis* may be called for to a degree distinctive to the psychiatry setting concerns not conflicts between particular virtues, of the kind just illustrated, but rather the setting as a whole. In this setting, as we have seen, a limited repertoire of actions is available to the practitioner. At least in traditional, Aristotelian conceptions, virtues are expressed in the form of deeds. Yet the deeds through which the practitioner can express her virtues in the psychiatry setting are limited: for the most part, they are words, body language, gestures, and demeanor. Granted, the currency of the healing exchange is meanings—if not entirely, then to a significant extent—and words, body language, gestures, and demeanor are all central vehicles of such a currency. Nonetheless, this is a limitation, we believe, that will call for a greater exercise of *phronesis* than would many other practices. Most virtues, and certainly most of the virtues called for by the psychiatry setting, include not only a range of actions but a much broader range of word, gesture or expression than are believed helpful to healing, or permitted by restrictions on the boundaries of the therapeutic relationship. In everyday life, for example, the expression of personal warmth is closely tied to bodily gesture, and actions writ large—so much so that without hugs, pats, and other contact, the body language of closeness, sympathy, and solidarity, the sincerity, or genuineness of one's warmth might be doubted. Yet, in the restrained setting of practice most of these grosser behavioral expressions are avoided, or actually proscribed.

Given the limitations imposed by this restricted behavioral and communicative repertoire, the practitioner must make every word, gesture and facial expression a telling one, every slightest response in this restrained space a communication of unmistakable and vibrant force. Moreover, as we saw earlier, patients' disorder will sometimes detract from their ability to receive (and give) communicatively, distorting the messages that are conveyed to them. In this difficult and limiting situation, it seems to us, knowing how to communicate effectively will require a remarkable degree of *phronesis* in practitioners.

Conclusion

The practitioner's virtues we selected for examination here were to serve several purposes. We wanted to emphasize how the demand for many everyday virtues such as trustworthiness and self-control, required in every imaginable situation, is magnified within psychiatric practice. Moreover, we wanted to show how the demands of the practice setting, and of the social role assigned to the psychiatrist, transform some traits that in ordinary contexts might have a very different meaning and moral significance. The trustworthiness, propriety, gender sensitivity, empathy, genuine personal warmth, self-knowledge, self-unity, integrity, hopeful patience, unselfing, realism, respectfulness, leadership, authenticity, and *phronesis* we have sketched were not intended to comprise a complete depiction of the character of the virtuous psychiatrist, however. As we emphasized at the start of this chapter, these traits were selected, primarily, because they each represented a distinctive kind of virtue, or a trait called for by distinctive features of the psychiatry setting—fulfilling our promise to eliminate the unsatisfactory vagueness adhering to talk of virtues by anchoring each to specifics of the setting. Additional traits not included here or barely mentioned—Beauchamp's "sensitivity,"—might be equally important and valuable, we readily concede.

Our goal was not the ambitious one of listing all the practitioner's virtues. And indeed, the elastic ways in which those heterogeneous clusters of dispositions and capabilities comprising particular virtues are named and identified, as this chapter should have demonstrated, would likely impede efforts to provide a truly comprehensive accounting of all role-constituted virtues. Nonetheless, we want again to emphasize, the sampling of virtues described here is merely a selection and makes no claim to any comprehensiveness.

6 Character and Social Role

Introduction

The role morality introduced earlier in this book nicely accommodates the apparent uniqueness of the ethics for psychiatric practice and the method by which the goal or good of such practice, together with aspects of the practice setting, allow us to ascertain some of the particular virtues of the practitioner. This kind of unexceptional role morality has been endorsed for its applicability to professions such as medicine, as we saw, and has been judged to be appropriately paired with a virtue framework emphasizing the character of the practitioner. It is a pairing with ancient roots, we add. Aristotle accepted Plato's assumption that different social groups have different roles and virtues.[1] But social roles for the Greeks, based as they were on differences perceived to be of nature and capability, were understood as preordained in a way quite different from more recent conceptions. (See MacIntyre 1984.)

Wedding social roles to an emphasis on the personal qualities of the practitioner in this way introduces some tensions, despite its apparent fit. At least as they are understood today, character and roles are in certain respects

[1] See Gorgias (1260a: 27–28).

antithetical. Not as immediately obvious, nor as troubling, within non-aretaic frameworks such as the Kantian and Utilitarian ones, these incompatibilities between character-based ethics and conceptions of social role are the broad focus of the present chapter. They can be eased, we conclude, but these tensions and their unsettling implications cannot be entirely expunged. They must first be clearly understood, however, and their relation to some misleading conceptions of social role, character, and behavior must be identified. We here emphasize a point previously acknowledged within professional ethics—that professional roles constitute part of the characterization identity of the practitioner. They are an integral part of who the person is conceived to be—by himself or herself, and by others. And, we shall see, they comprise part of the individual's normative "practical" identity (Korsgaard). Unlike some other social roles but in this respect like familial ones, professional roles are better described as inhabited than merely acted or played.

Important aspects of our ethical theory for psychiatric practice are held hostage by misunderstandings and misconceptions in this area it should be added, so this distinction is a significant one. In addition to these very broad questions about character and social role, we introduce a residue of related ethical concerns not explored thus far, each reflecting some aspect of the tension between the holistic notion of character and the segmented one of social roles. These include dilemmas and moral quandaries arising out of incompatible or dual roles, and the ethical status of inconstant virtues. In the second part of the chapter, we take up another group of issues that have arisen in various guises throughout the previous pages. These relate to the genuineness with which practitioner's responses are manifested and to the opportunity to feign such responses afforded by the combination of the practice-based model of virtue acquisition embraced here and certain aspects of the psychiatry setting. In assessing the moral status of seemingly virtuous responses that are actually feigned—whether because they are the initial efforts of learners, or because they reflect inevitable lapses from ideal practice—we return to the issue of how professional virtues are fostered. The moral philosophical distinction between semblances and counterfeits of virtue resolves some of the seeming incompatibility between an embrace of authenticity and wholeheartedness and the necessities of virtue learning. But here, as elsewhere in this book, we acknowledge the need for rules as well as virtues even if, finally, such rules are to be derived from those virtues.

Character and Roles as Antithetical

At the heart of any virtue theory is character, the unique and idiosyncratic construct that holds, and holds together, all the dispositions and traits making each individual the unique person, and moral agent, that he or she is. Like the notion of a person's identity (at least as traditionally conceived), that of character is understood as something enduring, defining, and integrated.[2] Rather than a succession of more fleeting states, "character" implies the existence of a collection of stable, long-term dispositions to act and respond in particular ways, traits definitive of the person possessing them. On this model, in Martha Nussbaum's words, "settled patterns of motive, emotion, and reasoning…lead us to call someone a person of a certain sort" (Nussbaum 1999: 170). Because in this conception of character there are inner states as well as their outer manifestations, a person may be seen to possess a *persona* (or several), which she projects out into the world. But character is not usually regarded as reducible to the *persona* (or *personae*): no *persona* will be more than superficial and potentially misleading appearances in contrast to the underlying structure that constitutes character.

These claims about character, and about the self's unity and identity, rest on metaphysical assumptions that we accept, although they will not be further defended here. (For an account of the metaphysical tenets involved, see, for example, Radden 1996.) However, we do not mean to suggest that this account is accurate in any empirically verifiable way (nor is the present work one of metaphysics). And indeed, much contemporary psychology and philosophy would challenge the coherence of such a picture of the self, with its emphasis on a core of traits that are relatively unchanging. (Those favoring the fragmentary and disputed subject of postmodernism would not accept this conception, for example, nor would social scientists critical of trait analyses, as we shall see presently.) But these are some of the metaphors that cling to the conception of character as it occurs in both classical and contemporary variants on virtue theory.[3]

Apparently antithetical to this conception of character are some presuppositions associated with the notion of social role. Such roles are rule-dictated

---

[2] Some of the difficulties of employing virtue concepts such as integrity with a fragmented, postmodern self are evident in recent work by Cox et al. (2003).

[3] While other moral theories may presuppose this account, they need not. In virtue theory, it is inescapable.

ways of responding in circumscribed social contexts. In Michael Hardimon's definition, which captures standard present day ideas, roles are described as, "constellations of institutionally specified rights and duties organized around an institutionally specified social function" (Hardimon 1994: 334). Implications of this definition include that (a) persons may adopt different roles with different social contexts ("functions"), (b) role incompatibilities may prevent a person's adopting some pairs of roles simultaneously, yet (c) people often inhabit multiple, compatible roles, sometimes simultaneously, sometimes sequentially. So understood, social roles seem to allow us to see the person as changing from role to role and setting to setting (or function to function), chameleon-like, and thus comprising no more than, and being potentially reducible to, a series of transformative *personae*. The tension, and question, then become apparent. How can a discourse of social roles capture the sense of character presupposed by virtue theory? Playing roles may perhaps be accommodated by an action-focused, deontological framework such as the traditional Kantian one. But it seems at odds with the conception of character underlying virtue theory.[4]

A vivid expression of this problem is found in the ideas about compartmentalization raised earlier. If the account proposed by MacIntyre is accurate, a moral danger attaches to understanding one's responses as merely role specific. It is a danger that extends to role morality more generally, and to the assumption that right conduct or particular virtues are role and context relative (both in the [weak] sense of imposing additional, role specific obligations, and in the more controversial [strong] sense of exempting the person from the demands of broad-based morality). The danger, as MacIntyre construes it, is that the individual will lose the ability to stand aside from particular roles and to evaluate and respond to situations as a human agent, *tout court*. In thus reducing the self to a sequence of role-constituted *personae*, that would be to jeopardize, or even expunge, the sense of oneself as an integrated moral and psychological whole, and place at risk one's status as a moral agent.

MacIntyre depicts the tension identified here as a product of post-Enlightenment times. Modernity, as he says, "partitions each human life into a variety of segments, each with its own norms and modes of behavior." When the individual and the roles that he plays are sharply separated, or

---

[4] To the extent that Kantianism is recast as character-based along the lines developed by Barbara Herman, it too will suffer from this apparent mismatch (Herman 1993).

when the different role—and quasi-role—enactments of an individual life are separated, "that life comes to appear as nothing but a series of unconnected episodes." So far from Aristotelian conceptions of character and the virtues are these effects that MacIntyre denies the self as thus conceived is "a bearer of the Aristotelian virtues," What are today called virtues are merely "professional *skills*, deployed in those situations where they can be effective" (MacIntyre 1980: 190–1, emphasis added).

So entirely contrary to MacIntyre's is our view, then, that we need not take issue with him on this last point. For rather than all virtues being demoted to mere professional skills, as MacIntyre describes, we believe that some professional skills can be construed as virtues. Nonetheless, MacIntyre may be right that changes in conceptions of the self and its roles occurring since the eighteenth century have sharpened the tension between roles and character. That, at least today, there is a tendency toward the kind of compartmentalization MacIntyre fears has been found through empirical study, moreover. Recently reviewed by John Doris, a considerable body of social psychology research appears to confirm a human tendency toward responses that are situation or role specific (Doris 2002). People's moral and altruistic behavior, in particular, have been shown to be more specific to particular situations and roles than we might have expected, and more specific than is presupposed in traditional philosophical conceptions of the enduring characteristics making up character.

Predictive and explanatory appeals to traits are familiar not only from virtue theory but from trait psychology as well, Doris reminds us. But he judges such appeals to be very often empirically inadequate, confounded, as he believes they are by "the extraordinary situational sensitivity observed in human behavior" (Doris 2002: 15). Virtues are supposed to be what trait theory names "robust" traits, that is, to display trait-relevant behavior across a wide variety of trait-relevant situations, even situations that are not conducive to such behavior (Doris 2002: 18). Yet evidence from social psychology instead supports a "situationist" view whereby trait-relevant behavior is surprisingly situation-specific. At best there are "socially sustained virtues," dispositions that will manifest themselves only when there is a properly constructed social environment. These are far from the all-weather, robust traits presupposed, and apparently required, by virtue theory. The problem with character explanations, then, Doris concludes, is that "They presuppose the existence of character structures that actual people do not often possess" (Doris 2002: 6).

Doris's conclusion is a qualified one, notice: not "never" but "do not often (possess)." And "do not," not "cannot (possess)." Thus, one way to read these findings, we suggest, is that they point to the need for greater efforts to counter our human situationist inclinations. Rather than refuting MacIntyre's claims, they might be thought to make all the more urgent MacIntyre's call for moral integrity as a remedy against role-segmented behavior.

To make good the case for character ethics against these empirical findings, however, we need to clarify the notion of playing a role in the context of role morality. What kinds of role are professional roles, it must be asked? What other social roles are they like? And what do the relations they bear to other social roles suggest about how to understand them?

Hardimon's analysis of social roles is again helpful as we explore these questions (Hardimon 1994). Here, contractual roles are distinguished from noncontractual roles. The first are entered into voluntarily, the second come with birth. Although less common, these latter, noncontractual, roles are not less important, Hardimon emphasizes. Our very ethical identity, as he puts it, is shaped by "the social arrangements into which we are born" (Hardimon 1994: 353). We will return to this matter of ethical identity presently, but to emphasize that it must not be construed as, or as merely, a function of the noncontractual aspect of those roles that come with birth. Like many roles, professional roles are contractual rather than noncontractual. But that by no means precludes their being identity conferring.

In a first try to find appropriate analogies for professional roles, we naturally turn to theatrical ones. And an explicit comparison has been made between those adopting professional roles and stage actors: Andrew Crowden notes that when an actor plays the part of a friend, for example, it will be both like and unlike real friendship, just as is true with professional-client relationships (Crowden 2003). There are other similarities between professional and stage roles as well; each is contractual, for example, on Hardimon's classification. Yet the analogy between professional and theatrical roles is limited at best, we believe, and these similarities superficial and potentially misleading. Stage actors adopt many parts in many plays and, because of this, their roles are not in any permanent way part of their identity[5]; moreover, to perform those parts they abide by rules, but these are not moral rules. (Also, social norms appear to restrict dramatic performance to its context. In everyday life off the stage, expressions such as "he's (just) acting," "she's playing a part,"

---

[5] A tendency to play roles may be part of their identity, of course; presumably it is central to the nature of professional actors.

"more histrionics," have a ring that seems to mark the acted or played role as undesirably inauthentic.)

The dissimilarities between theatrical and professional roles encourage us to search for stronger analogies. And indeed there are such, we want now to insist—in familial roles. Some of the more permanent roles we inhabit are these familial ones: parental roles, sibling roles, offspring roles, and so on. These roles, or many of them, are instances of Hardimon's noncontractual roles, coming by dint of birth. (Since it can be the result of a decision to bear or adopt children, the role of parent looks to be an intermediate case, alerting us that the distinction between contractual and noncontractual roles is not exclusive.) In this respect then, most familial roles are dissimilar to professional roles, which are entirely contractual.

Yet familial roles actually have the two earlier noted characteristics absent from stage roles, and these similarities are shared with professional roles. They confer identity, and they generate role specific moral demands. And these similarities, we want to emphasize, are more significant than any differences between familial and professional roles.

Familial roles confer or even partly constitute characterization identity: I am a mother; I do not play the role of mother. As a mother I cannot "play" (the part of) a mother, except perhaps on stage, or screen. Outside of the theatrical context, merely acting a part is associated with acting without authenticity, or without the sincerity and wholeheartedness usually deemed appropriate, as we noted; indeed, "merely acting" suggests something close to intentional deception practiced for ignoble reasons. In acknowledging this contrast, it seems useful to propose that to varying degrees roles may be either played or they may be integrated into personal identity. These latter can be said to be "inhabited." Inhabiting the identity-conferring role of mother, I do not, and cannot (except in the special theatrical context) play it. Because professional roles are similarly identity constituting, they are also inhabited rather than merely played. (There may be intermediate cases between these two kinds of roles, we add, as there may be between familial and nonfamilial roles, and professional and nonprofessional ones. But both familial and professional roles come in easily recognized paradigms and are clear-cut instances of inhabiting rather than playing roles.) The full moral import of the distinction between playing and inhabiting roles will be explored presently.

The second similarity between professional and familial roles is that they each generate role specific moral and ethical obligations. My parental duties to my children are different, and greater, than those to others' children just as, we saw earlier, the physician's relationship to his patients includes responsibilities, attitudes, and demands different from and greater than any he may have to strangers.

If the analogy with parental roles is apt, then—except when participating in theatrical performance—it can be no more possible for a doctor to merely play or act the part of doctor than it is for a person who is a parent to play or act that part. And just as a person who is a mother cannot play or act being a mother because she *is* a mother, so by analogy, we want to insist that this doctor does not play or act being a doctor, she *is* a doctor. Doctors inhabit their professional roles, which form part of their (characterization) identity—and also, we will now explain, part of their more explicitly normative identity.

The identity conferring aspect of roles and their normative implications have also been explored by Hardimon. He defines "role identification" as (i) occupying the role; (ii) recognizing that one occupies the role; and (iii) conceiving of oneself as someone for whom the norms of the role function as reasons. As he puts it, "The process of coming to identify with a social role is at once a process of coming to regard certain considerations as reasons and…of coming to conceive of oneself as a person of a certain kind" (Hardimon 1994: 357–358). People identify this way with their roles and gain from them reasons, including moral reasons, for carrying out the tasks of these roles. Hardimon provides an example: that of the man who identifies with the role of father, "the fact that he is a father provides him with a reason—a moral reason—for caring for his children" (Hardimon 1994: 362). Further explication and grounding for these ideas can be found within contemporary moral philosophy. Christine Korsgaard, for example, allows us to see how moral reasons emerge from identity-conferring roles. Possessing a conception of ourselves, something like what we have called here self or characterization identity, she reminds us, is a consequence of the structure of self-consciousness. She names that conception "practical" identity, defined as a description under which you find your life to be worth living and your actions to be worth undertaking (Korsgaard 1996: 101). This conception is the source of (moral) reasons and obligations, and thus normative.[6]

---

[6] Thus "Reflective distance from our impulses makes it both possible and necessary to decide which ones we will act on: it forces us to act for reasons. At the same time, and relatedly, it forces us to have a conception of our own identity, a conception which identifies us with the source of those reasons" (Korsgaard 1996: 113).

So in inhabiting their professional roles, we want to add, doctors find reasons, including moral reasons, for carrying out their professional duties. Roles that are thus inhabited form part of their normative, "practical" identity. Moreover, the features of the psychiatry setting (such as patient vulnerabilities) that, as we have put it, "call for" certain virtues in practitioners, might equally be said to be *moral reasons for the practitioner to acquire those virtues*. These identity constituting, and moral reason conferring, aspects of professional roles have been recognized to apply across the professions, it should be added. Of lawyer's roles, David Luban has written that commitments to the duties of a profession can be, and frequently are, "among the deepest loyalties and commitments in our lives" (Luban 1984: 142).

Summing up then, we have argued that strong analogies link professional and familial roles, even though the first are contractual, while the second are often not. Both kinds of roles are identity conferring, each bringing with it specific moral implications in the form of moral reasons for particular responses. Because of the way we are personally and morally entrenched in, and identify with, these roles, it is more accurate to speak of our inhabiting, rather than acting or playing, them.

Although we have demonstrated that doctors, like mothers, inhabit their roles, there is one notable qualification on this assertion to which we will return later in this chapter. Whether we speak of professional or parental roles, when the new role is first acquired, or imposed, through training programs in the one case, and the birth or adoption of a child in the other, the fledgling doctors or mothers may not yet experience themselves as inhabiting the role. Instead they may seem to themselves to play the part, enacting it without any accompanying sense of authenticity. ("This is not really me," they might even feel, or "I hope no-one sees through me" [Rosenthal 2003].) Adopting the conduct and appearance of an ethical doctor, or mother, may have to precede feeling like a doctor, or mother.

We can now return to the studies Doris describes, which he considers supportive of a "situationist" view whereby trait-relevant behavior usually thought to bespeak the presence of all-weather, robust virtues is actually surprisingly situation-specific. Our first point is that because social roles differ in the important ways noted, the situation specificity of people's responses must reflect the kinds of situation, and role, involved. Because professional (and family) roles are identity conferring, for example, traits associated with the adoption of those roles can be expected to be less likely to engender situation-specific responses. And indeed, Doris concedes at least of one set of responses usually supposed to result from a person's enduring moral character and identity: helping behavior among friends, family, and coworkers. People help most, and are most helped by, the ones they know and love—when, as he puts it, "social ties exist" (Doris 2002: 35). And if we are more inclined to help intimates and acquaintances than strangers, it will surely be because our roles of friend, sibling, or even coworker are permanent or relatively so, and to that extent more likely to be identity conferring ones—or, alternatively put, because we care more about them.

Speaking generally of "situationism," we want to point out that if the tendency toward situation-specific responses is part of our shared human nature, and an ongoing tendency and temptation, then a strong and virtuous moral character, together with the appropriate support provided by what Doris calls a "properly constructed social environment," could be proof against it. Our aim in this book has been to analyze the ingredients of the first, and set in place some of the groundwork for the second.

In addition, we believe that with its focus on ideals rather than circumscribed rights, wrongs, and duties, a virtue-based ethics is well equipped to counter the tendency toward situation-specific moral responses. Achieving an entirely virtuous moral character may be beyond reach for almost everyone, an ideal toward which, because of our situationist tendencies, we inevitably fall short in our strivings. But if so, then virtue theory provides a language for identifying, understanding, and teaching, such striving, and our efforts to reach that ideal. Doris himself concludes something very close to this, acknowledging the possibility that attempting to emulate a virtuous "exemplar," as he says "is the most effective way to facilitate ethically desirable conduct" (Doris 2002: 149). Efforts to habituate more robust virtues mindful of these temptations, he believes, will best allow us to overcome the tendency toward situationism. "Only by being aware of the situational threats to responsibility can we act as responsible persons in as many situations as possible" (Doris 2002: 153).

Compartmentalization and Incompatible Roles

The inner, moral psychological analogue of the measurable behavior Doris terms "situationism" is found in MacIntyre's compartmentalized individual. Equipped with the distinction between acting or playing and inhabiting professional roles we can now return to MacIntyre's concerns. Only through the cultivation of integrity (and constancy) could compartmentalization be avoided by the person working within large bureaucratic structures, MacIntyre has argued. And certainly, we have seen, such virtues are important for the ethical practitioner. She inhabits her role of psychiatrist, rather than merely acting or playing; thus the practitioner defines herself in terms of the professional integrity it requires of her. And the identity conferring or constituting aspect of professional roles means that, as we saw earlier, these roles are not able to be "put on or off like a suit of clothes." So the practitioner who inhabits a professional role rather than merely acting or playing it will also be some proof against compartmentalization. Whatever the temptation to compartmentalize imposed by the strongly differentiated demands of some settings, her knowledge of who she is, a psychiatrist, will serve to extend and enhance the robustness of her moral responses.

Difficult cases of role conflict, which also seem likely to induce compromising forms of compartmentalization, are not distinctive to the bureaucratized settings MacIntyre describes. What are known as dual roles or double agency occur in a range of other settings as well. Wherever, in order to fulfill the goals of some practice, profession, or institution, the practitioner is expected to at the least add to and balance, and at most to set aside, the goals and goods of her own professional practice, dual roles—and so potential role conflict—are involved.

One instance of dual roles was introduced earlier in this book. The goal of public safety imposes a special duty on psychiatrists in the commitment of those whose disorder renders them dangerous to themselves or others. In ordering involuntary seclusion and treatment, the practitioner must look beyond the individual patient toward the community. Here, the broader goal of public safety may be relatively easy to reconcile with the narrower one of healing the individual patient. Civil commitment is widely, and we believe reasonably, regarded as in the interests of dangerous patients. It provides them with much needed treatment, prevents them from committing criminal acts for which they might receive harsh punishment, for example, and saves them from personal harm. Patient interests and public safety appear to be compatible ends, in this case, and a broadly paternalistic and protective principle can be seen to govern both individual treatment and civil commitment. It was argued earlier that uncommon virtue will be demanded of the practitioner because of the morally hazardous power entrusted in him with the duty of civil commitment. But, while imposing an additional role on the practitioner, this duty does not usually impose strongly incompatible dual roles.

More controversial cases of incompatible—and so morally troubling—dual roles occur in the practice of psychiatry when, for instance, the additional and potentially competing goals and goods are those of for-profit delivery systems, the military, and the justice system. These situations of competing and potentially incompatible ideals and goals that seem to impose role conflicts occur in managed care medicine when the doctor is expected to be both healer and gate-keeper, it has often been emphasized. Such dual roles have been construed as requiring sacrifice of the individual patient's health for the health of the collective, and, sometimes, even for transparently economic, marketplace goals of the company. Military psychiatry during wartime offers additional examples of role conflict. Here, practitioners are asked to restore their patients to fighting readiness with recognition that the goal of national defense may be inimical to healing or to the present (or future) psychic well-being of the individual soldier.[7] The forensic psychiatrist, too, will be required to set aside the goal of healing in order to evaluate a defendant's psychological status: his fitness to stand trial, for instance, or readiness to receive punishment. And when serving the end of justice this way is judged incompatible with serving a commitment to healing, role conflict will occur. Practitioners required to medicate death row prisoners to achieve a state of sanity so that execution can take place have argued that their proper role of caring for the prisoner's health cannot be reconciled with the judicial ends of adjudication and punishment. (See Freedman and Halpern 1996; Freedman and Radden 2006.)

Two different theoretical approaches have attempted to avoid the conclusion that the roles imposed by forensic practice must place the psychiatrist in moral or ethical jeopardy. In a controversial discussion Paul Appelbaum resolves the apparently conflicting roles imposed on forensic psychiatrists by insisting that the paramount goals and goods of forensic practice are not the same as those adhered to by other practitioners in psychiatry (Appelbaum

---

[7] Such a conflict of roles is evident in the following description by journalist Dan Baum, who writes that in the war with Iraq in 2003, "an Army staff sergeant, disturbed by the sight of an Iraqi's mutilated body, confided his concern to his unit's combat-stress officer and, according to the Army, asked to be sent back to the United States. He was charged with cowardly conduct. (The charge was subsequently reduced to dereliction of duty and ultimately dismissed.) Although this was an extremely unusual case, military psychiatrists agree that their first job is to keep soldiers fighting. Even when a soldier is on the verge of cracking up, 'if he's more a benefit to the unit than a detriment,' the Defense Department psychiatrist Thomas Burke told me, an Army shrink's job is to 'get him back to duty'." (Baum 2004: 49).

1997). To the extent that these apparent incompatibilities exist within forensic psychiatry, justice, truthfulness and respect for persons must be valued and honored above personal obligations of beneficence and nonmaleficence. (See also Strasburger et al. 1997.) The forensic psychiatrist chooses to wear a judicial hat.

In contrast, Philip Candilis, Richard Martinez and Christina Dording have tried to reconcile forensic practice with traditional, dyadic patient-professional values; balancing two hats, they argue, is not only possible, but right (Candilis et al. 2001). Most professionals manage to accommodate and reconcile their potentially incompatible personal values with their professional values, it is pointed out. The same accommodation requires that the pull toward "therapeutic relationship" can and should be acknowledged alongside that of "expert role." The division of functions, "an expert in one place, a clinician in another, a complete person at home" is not consistent with the particulars of human drama and the holistic manner in which most of us experience our lives. Such an approach "fails to capture the richness" of lived experience (Candilis et al. 2001: 172–173). In forensic work, it is not possible, or desirable, to detach forensic consultations from traditional commitments to patients, they insist.

Candilis, Martinez, and Dording are surely right that with a recognition and insistence that their personal and several professional obligations constitute equally valuable parts of their identity that cannot be entirely relinquished in the forensic setting, practitioners may be effective in humanizing that setting and reconciling apparently conflicting roles. Yet stark cases will remain, such as the one they provide when the practitioner is both therapist and forensic expert for the same individual, or the one noted above where the psychiatrist is asked to impose medication to ready a prisoner for execution. Here, at least, Appelbaum's uncompromising implication is correct: the practitioner cannot wear both hats.

At the very least, we believe, two conditions must be met if the practitioner undertaking these dual roles is to avoid morally corrupting internal divisions. One is that the ends or goals of each role are themselves morally justified and embraced, as such, by the practitioner. The second is that, by habituating the self-knowledge and psychological self-unity seen to be its preconditions, as well as engaging in consultation with others, the virtue of integrity is cultivated.

In his account of this sort of requirement, Hardimon demands that a social role itself be "reflectively acceptable," when "Determining whether a given role is reflectively acceptable involves stepping back from that role in thought and asking whether it is a role people ought to occupy and play ... judging that it is ... meaningful, rational, or good" (Hardimon 1994: 348). Role conflicts were shown to arise in three kinds of practice: civil commitment, wartime psychiatry, and forensic psychiatry. (We return to the example of the managed care setting below.) The goals and goods of each of these—public safety, national security, and justice, respectively, are all unexceptional ends. Merely as a citizen and a responsible human being, the practitioner likely accepts such broad-based values. And each role seems to meet Hardimon's standard of reflective acceptability.

Arguably, the difference between forensic or wartime psychiatry, and managed care psychiatry, is considerable. The means may be another matter, but few would question the judicial and public safety goals of forensic psychiatry, or even the national security goals of wartime psychiatry; in contrast, few would not question the goals of managed care delivery systems to the extent that they are solely construed as maximizing company profits.[8] But the advent of managed care systems has also seen new recognition of the broader societal interests at stake in health care and of duties that involve not only fiduciary concerns but medical stewardship over limited resources (Sabin 1994, 1995). The goals and values of managed care systems can be understood in several ways; but as responsible concern over fair resource allocation and stewardship, they will also be reflectively acceptable to many.

Yet, just as there may be practitioners who embrace as morally justified and reflectively acceptable the goals of managed care companies, whether construed as "profit-seeking" or "fair resource allocation," or both, so there will be those who resist some of the means or methods by which public safety, justice, and or national security are affected. And to the extent that her conscience forbids any of these practices or rejects such ends, or means—the practitioner who has a moral objection to capital punishment, or to war, for

[8] As it arises in business ethics, the "role problem" involves squaring the amoral or nonmoral (profit-maximizing) goals of business with the ethics demanded of its practitioners (Swanton 2007: 210). Christine Swanton's solution is to distinguish "prototype" virtues from role virtues, and to insist that the more general, and vague, role-undifferentiated prototype virtues must serve to inhibit the headlong pursuit of institutional goals. Since medicine and psychiatry are "good" professions in the sense that their goals and goods have unquestionable moral value, appeal to prototype virtues may have little applications for psychiatry, however. Even in the managed care setting, the regulative ideals of the professional will serve as constraints on the pursuit of any amoral goals.

instance—will have internal divisions jeopardizing her moral integrity. She must, and must be permitted to, refuse to adopt the hat of forensic or military psychiatrist, respectively.

What then of the practitioner with no such qualms? At the least, we believe, the moral dangers involved in wearing two hats must be acknowledged. The practitioner who has donned the hat of the forensic or military psychiatrist without recognizing the tension incumbent in the role should strenuously seek moral integrity. Achieving such integrity will involve habituating the traits of self-knowledge and psychological self-unity which, we saw earlier, are some of its central preconditions, and resisting internal compartmentalization by engaging in dialogue and consultation with others.

Inconstant Virtue

Spurred by the findings Doris notes that emphasize the situation- and role-specific nature of much actual ethical behavior, we must now consider another kind of incomplete virtue and moral danger: inconstant virtue. What of those role-constituted and identity-constituting virtues whose manifestations are inconsistently displayed, or are perhaps even limited to the context of practice? If the trustworthy practitioner were to show untrustworthiness in his nonprofessional relationships, are these professional displays of trustworthiness in some way morally incomplete? Arguably, a person who exhibits such inconstant virtue cannot be said to truly possess the virtue. Followers of John McDowell, for example, might insist that possession of real trustworthiness would be incompatible with such inconstant virtue: to be trustworthy guarantees being fully trustworthy (McDowell 1979). In light of the evidence Doris brings to bear, however, such a stance seems to fly in the face of a predictable scenario: the case of the inconstantly virtuous practitioner, capable of and given to genuinely manifesting a virtue in one setting, but reluctant or negligent about manifesting it in others. The professionally trustworthy practitioner who is unfaithful to a spouse is one example; the practitioner who would never lie to a patient but submits fraudulent income tax returns may be another.

This issue does not apply to all the virtues of the good psychiatrist, it should be stressed, since several of these are, as virtues, dependent on the setting. The practitioner whose ability to manifest the role-constituted virtue of unselfing, for example, may not find use or value for that trait elsewhere. Indeed, as we emphasized earlier, the preference for mutuality of exchange in everyday life might make unselfing a socially inappropriate and imprudent response outside of the professional setting. The practitioner who exhibits exquisitely tuned unselfing in the clinic and is socially clumsy and insensitive elsewhere does not show inconstant virtue. But trustworthiness, as well as several other virtues called for by the psychiatry setting, are everyday virtues, demanded as much in nonprofessional as in professional life. The possession of these virtues, at least, runs the risk of being inconstantly exhibited.

Remaining with our example of inconstant trustworthiness, there are several preliminary points to make (though none is sufficient to entirely resolve the problem). First, to the extent that this is real trustworthiness at all, practitioners given to such inconstant virtue will be rarer than we might otherwise expect due to the identity constituting aspect of professional roles. This, we recognize, is finally an empirical matter. But because these are roles that are often inhabited rather thoroughly and deeply and not merely acted or played, the practitioner who has sought to habituate trustworthiness in professional settings must be expected to exhibit that virtue in other parts of his life. Moreover, following the Aristotelian model by which virtues are habituated through practice, the presence of trustworthiness in the practice setting might be expected to penetrate his other roles, eventually affecting his everyday life responses as well. Inconstant trustworthiness may be expected to occur, but infrequently.

When it does occur, such inconstant trustworthiness will indicate the kind of moral flaw, and moral danger of which MacIntyre has warned. The divided person jeopardizes the virtue of moral integrity (which, emphasizing precisely the quality of reliability at issue here, MacIntyre sometimes also calls "constancy"). By its nature such moral integrity is, like *phronesis*, a kind of meta virtue, a trait concerned not so much with different settings or actions as with the relationship between one's other virtues, and the wholeness and coherence of one's moral character. The practitioner whose trustworthiness is inconstant lacks moral integrity.

Moral integrity may occur in varying degrees, certainly. (See Cox et al. 2003). Virtues are ideals, and goals; we fall somewhat short of reaching all of them. The practitioner who exhibits inconstant trustworthiness, or warmth, or patience, or any of the virtues of practice, is not entirely vicious, he is partially virtuous. Yet because the temptations toward inconstant virtues must be acknowledged, we here suggest, some minimal standards should perhaps be invoked, employing the action-guiding rules of non-aretaic ethics. A supremely or ideally virtuous practitioner will manifest the virtue of trustworthiness (and every other virtue) in every setting. But a minimal ethical standard closer to those found in the do's and dont's of ethical codes for practice may require considerably less. At the least, the virtue must be consistently manifested within the practice setting, and the practitioner should recognize the importance of unifying and integrating his moral life.

Learning Virtues through Habituation

The transformation from trainee to full professional, we have seen, can be understood through emphasis on the transformation of self-identity that allows identity conferring and constituting roles such as familial and professional roles to be inhabited rather than merely enacted. Here, in the concept of self-identity, is the link between social roles and role-constituted virtues. The practitioner who has become a professional, we saw, not only occupies the role but recognizes that she does. Her role, then, will have become part of her self- or characterization identity. Moreover, she will conceive of herself as a person for whom the norms of the role, its regulative ideals, in Oakley and Cocking's language, function as moral reasons. Her self-identity will include not only the recognition "I am a psychiatrist," but acknowledgment of the norms of her role "These responses are morally incumbent upon me" or "These features of the setting are moral reasons for me to act." When the practitioner becomes a psychiatrist, the virtues suitable to his role will be a core part of his character and identity.[9] The way social roles become inhabited and virtues are habituated have bearing on questions about the moral status of virtue acquisition.

How are virtues instilled? The short answer to that question offered already in this book is Aristotle's: by habituation. The moral education of which Aristotelian spoke in the *Nichomachean Ethics* was that for a young Athenian man making his way toward an adulthood of nobility and justice, however. Its applicability to the question of how the role-constituted virtues of psychiatric practice described in Chapter 5 are to be acquired by young adults entering the profession, remains to be established.

---

[9] For a fuller account of the relation between self-identity and moral character, see Taylor 1992, Flanagan and Rorty 1990.

Aristotle's emphasis on practice and habituation was a response to Socrates' overly cognitivist conception of virtue as a form of knowledge. Aristotle instead insisted that the sources of virtue were emotional as well as cognitive and began in practice and in a kind of "learning by doing" that would only later allow the beginner to recognize the reason why what is noble and just is so, and value it for its own sake. Thus the ultimate end toward which the beginner's practice is aimed is "that he should become the sort of person who does virtuous things in full knowledge of what he is doing, choosing to do them for their own sake, and acting out of a settled state of character" (1105a: 28–33). The starting point for this kind of training is a person who *already recognizes, and recognizes the value of, virtuous actions;* time and practice will enhance his enjoyment of doing them (Burnyeat 1980: 69). (The ingredients of that starting point, as Aristotle knew, began much earlier, in childhood and youth. The emergence of young adults with appropriate moral responses toward others, as contemporary moral development theorists suggest, probably requires some native "prosocial" inclinations that have been carefully shaped and "induced" [Hoffman] through moral education. [See, for example, Hoffman 2000.])

Further understanding of how this emphasis on practice could help when we think of instilling the role-constituted virtues of a practice such as psychiatry also comes from Greek philosophical traditions wherein the different sciences were classified according to their methods, subject matter, relation to theory, and such features. Aristotle recognized that medicine was not only a theoretical science but a practical one. Aspects of the uncodifiability of medical knowledge and its practical orientation meant that medicine was to be learned through doing, both practicing, but also, Aristotle emphasizes, by observing the practice of those more experienced.

The moral education required for those training in psychiatry, then, will be guided by these two aspects of practice, repeated exercise of the capabilities and subcapabilities making up particular virtues, together with paying attention to the behavior of exemplary models. (Such models may be fictional and historical as well as actual, as those engaged in bioethics education rightly recognize.) Eventually, such virtues will become a kind of second nature, so deeply embedded in their possessor's character that they are like other good habits. But at first, we can imagine, they will be displayed in a clumsy and halting way, and will not be fully internalized. Like the youth already appreciative of the Athenian virtues of nobility and justice, the trainee practitioners will bring to this learning process a general appreciation, theoretical as well as affective. They will see the value of the character traits that will become their role-constituted practitioner's virtues. But only after much practice will they be able to exercise these virtues in full knowledge of what they are doing, as Aristotle says, choosing to do them for their own sake, and acting out of a settled state of character.

One aspect of the heterogeneity of the many role-constituted virtues described in the preceding pages has been demonstrated through emphasis on the different ways we can approach their habituation. As we saw, some very key practitioner's virtues appear unruly in the sense of requiring habituation that is indirect: what must be practiced, when it comes to habituating empathic responses, will be cognitive skills of perception, attention, and imagination. Habituating other virtues, in contrast, will be more direct. (Again, it is presupposed here that the trainee is a young adult possessed of the usual virtues and prosocial sensitivities as the result of moral education and competent parenting in childhood and youth.) Practicing trustworthiness will involve practicing behaving in a trustworthy way; practicing patience—responding patiently; practicing propriety—paying great attention to appearances, and so on. These latter virtues, acquired through practice in the most straightforward Aristotelian manner by practicing doing what they involve doing or responding the way they involve responding, are the concern of the following discussion. We return to the more complex matter of cultivating unruly virtues, such as enhanced empathy, in the concluding chapter of this book.

Feigning while Learning Virtues

The role-constituted virtue of hopefulness will serve as our particular example here. We want the practitioner to be a hopeful person, not merely to feign hopefulness in her professional role as a psychiatrist. We want hopefulness to be part of her character and identity, not a mere show. Yet if acquiring virtues involves habituation and practice, there must be incompletely achieved responses along the way. Granted, some initial advantage may be unlearned—she who brings a sanguine and optimistic temperament will more readily habituate the virtue of hopefulness, perhaps. Aiming to become a hopeful character will involve closely observing and trying to emulate the hopefulness exhibited by exemplary models, as well as employing cognitive and perceptual abilities to see reasons for hopefulness. But it will also involve striving to convey hopefulness, through gesture, expression, body language, speech, and other action. Thus, as these descriptions suggest, an ethics education based on the idea of a virtuous psychiatrist must depend on the internalization of at least some virtues that were initially adopted in appearance only. In instilling the virtues, it seems, there can be expected to be feelings and inner states not yet possessed, which the trainee must sometimes feign. In their recent discussion of clinical empathy, Larson and Yao explore the contrast outlined here when they distinguish "deep" from "surface" acting (Larson and Yao 2005). Surface acting involves "forging empathic behavior toward the patient, absent of consistent emotional and cognitive reactions," that is, it is *feigning an empathic response*. The preferred deep acting, which they analogize to the method-acting approach employed by some stage and screen actors, is described as "generating empathy consistent emotional and cognitive reactions before and during empathic interactions with the patient" (Larson and Yao 2005: 1100).

As we saw in Chapter 5, some virtues can readily be feigned in the psychiatry setting and, since it is incompatible with the desired authenticity, genuineness, and wholeheartedness that should attach to the expression of any virtues, such feigning seems to present an ethical problem for the practitioner. But how much of a problem this is, we must now determine.

What is the moral status of feigning when it is part of the process of habituation? Arguably, it will be ineffectual and thus not conducive to the goals and goods of practice. On the interpretation of Aristotle associated with McDowell, no virtue could ever be successfully feigned. Beauchamp seems to adopt this position, in the discussion introduced in Chapter 3, when he asserts that whenever the feelings, concerns, and attitudes of others are the morally relevant matters only the possession of certain virtues (his examples are human warmth and sensitivity) will "lead a person to notice what should be done" (Beauchamp 1999). Without genuine sensitivity or warmth, a practitioner would have insufficient awareness of what responses a particular situation called for to be able to feign the virtues required.

There is some force to this view in the example of sensitivity Beauchamp provides. By side-stepping a painful topic out of the misplaced delicacy of insincere or feigned sensitivity, a practitioner may miss an important disclosure from the patient, for example, nothing less than a genuine sensitivity and real delicacy could permit the sure-footed response the situation demands. Perhaps finally, real compassion, warmth, and sensitivity will always bring about the most effective healing. Nonetheless, this argument does not provide us with grounds for entirely condemning the feigning of virtues, just grounds for preferring genuine responses because of their added effectiveness.

Now of course it is generally true that the cultivation of virtues should serve to prevent deception, falsity, and counterfeit responses, rather than inviting them, and such feigning and pretending could be expected to corrupt the character of the practitioner, adding to it the vices of deception and dishonesty. The notion of feigned and faked "virtues" seems antithetical to any account of virtue and character derived from virtue theory. Such feigning also seems to contravene Kantian rules on how we can treat other people.[10] The patient is manipulated and deceived, manipulation and deception are both doubly wrong because this patient is already vulnerable to exploitation. And manipulating and deceiving the patient even if it is for her own good, is contrary to treating her, and the healing project, with appropriate respect.

But if feigning responses is an inescapable part of habituating virtues, how are we to view it? And indeed, how do we weigh any actual effectiveness of some feigned virtues (such as feigned patience, for example) against the apparent wrongfulness of deceiving patients in this way? To answer these questions and to resolve the morally problematic implication of our account of virtue acquisition that it invites, permits and perhaps even calls for, the feigning of virtues requires a more fine-grained analysis of feigning, pretending, and hypocrisy.

Semblances and Counterfeits of Virtue

Hypocrisy is a vice, it is widely agreed.[11] It involves dissembling about motives or practicing deception in order to appear in a favorable light and or further one's selfish interests.[12] This immediately seems to set true hypocrisy apart

[10] For a useful discussion of hypocrisy and consequentialism, see Szabados and Soifer (2004). When hypocrisy is used as a test against which to evaluate moral theories, these authors conclude, consequentialism does better than others.

[11] How bad a vice, is debatable. Szabados and Soifer, for instance, suggest that the extreme viciousness of hypocrisy emerges only with Judeo-Christian morality that "aimed to discount appearance and accent the state of one's inner soul (the inner, what God sees)" in a way quite alien to Aristotelian thinking (Szabados and Soifer 2004: 83).

[12] For fuller discussions of hypocrisy, see Crisp and Cowton 1994, McKinnon, 1991, 1999 and Szabados and Soifer 2004.

from the cases where a practitioner feigns virtues in the interests of healing or in order to learn the art of healing. Consider the following case of feigning virtue.

> Dr. K is seeing her patient for the first time after he has been hospitalized and medicated against his wishes. Angrily and wordily, her patient recounts an incident from his hospital stay about which, unbeknownst to him, Dr. K has been informed. Dr. K has some issues to think over before seeing her next patient, and finds herself distractedly musing over them instead of listening to a tale she already knows. Crossing her hands and straightening her back to give at least the body language of full attention, she feigns listening to his narrative.

Dr. K makes a show of listening to her patient in order to foster his trust in her, and his belief in her concern and caring; she does so without any personal or selfish motivation whatsoever. If not blameless, deceptions such as Dr. K's nonetheless cannot be equated with hypocrisy. Because motives create morally significant differences in such cases, it will be helpful to turn to a distinction found in scholastic and also in Confucian traditions (particularly the writing of Mencius), between semblances and counterfeits of virtue. There are "semblances" of virtue (acting virtuously not out of virtue but for some good end) but also "counterfeits" (affecting virtue for an ignoble end). And while semblances of virtue are recognized to be less valuable than the possession of real virtues in both Thomistic and Confucian traditions, semblances of virtue are granted some degree of moral worth (Yearley 1990: 19–23; 124–129). Guided by this analysis, we propose that even Dr. K, who feigns attentiveness to establish or maintain the therapeutic alliance, offers a semblance of that trait. She exhibits an ethical position distinguishable from that of the hypocritical practitioner who counterfeits patience for some transparently personal gain (a wish to feel powerful and in control, for example).

Counterfeiting virtues will always be unacceptable. Affecting a semblance of virtues, in contrast, is a consequence of adopting this account of the moral life. Instilling virtues not already ingrained in the character must depend on the internalization of at least some traits initially adopted in appearance only, that is, it must depend on semblances of virtue.

The motive-based distinction between semblances of virtue and counterfeited virtues allows us to see that semblances of virtue may be relatively benign faults. Nonetheless, more needs be said about what "good ends" will count as minimally acceptable motivation. Not every semblance undertaken for the patient's good, or the goal of healing, can be acceptable. The tricks and "pious frauds" practiced on patients in the past, raised in Chapter 5, are a vivid reminder of the dangers of well-intended, but unwarranted, pretenses. The position we believe appropriate, given the moral dangers of even semblances of virtue, is that any such semblances other than those affected while, and necessary to, learning virtues, will be better avoided. Dr. K owed her patient her full attention, and even her semblance of virtue was not entirely acceptable.

The feigning of virtues involved in acquiring them seems to be an unavoidable aspect of adopting a virtue-based approach to practice. At best, then, the dangers associated with such feigning of virtues can be recognized and acknowledged. And the trainee's progress in habituating virtues must be monitored and discussed in a supervisory setting, where the goal of fully habitual and more authentic responses can be kept in sight.

Conclusion

Some of the tensions, theoretical and practical, incumbent in the virtue-based system of professional role morality were explored here. These tensions can be properly evaluated, we have shown, only by emphasizing that professional roles, rather like familial ones, are inhabited, not merely acted or played: such roles constitute part of the "practical" identity of the practitioner. This alone takes us some distance in understanding the particular moral dangers of role conflict and inconstant virtues. When virtues, including the virtue of moral integrity, constitute part of a clinician's abiding practical identity or moral character, the inclination to tolerate conflicting or dual roles or to exhibit inconstant virtue will be lessened.

While also illuminated by philosophical explication, some of these difficulties—particularly those associated with inconstant virtues—were shown to require resolution through appeal to non-aretaic ethics. Rules can provide minimally acceptable levels of conduct when virtue ideals are not enough.

The second issue raised in this chapter brought together the model of virtue acquisition that is presupposed in the broadly Aristotelian account we have adopted, and concerns over the important role-constituted virtue of authenticity, described in Chapter 5. To effect their habituation, virtues must be practiced. And an inescapable part of that practice, for those instilling virtues or cultivating greater virtue, seems to include feigned responses. Thus mere "semblances" of virtue must precede real virtue as practitioners acquire the character of the virtuous psychiatrist. Although not the worst of moral weaknesses, these semblances of virtue are a danger for the practitioner and one only acceptable within the educational setting, we concluded, where close supervision provides trainees with a reminder of the limitations and deficiencies of semblances of virtue and the potential ethical danger they bring.

7 Case Studies in Psychiatric Virtues

Introduction

The cases in the following chapter serve several interrelated purposes. The first concerns the perspective from which such material is presented. Case material in bioethics, and also, indeed, the cases introduced thus far in this volume, are customarily written in the third person, and from an omniscient point of view. In this respect, they violate some of the basic insights from narrative theory highlighted in Tod Chambers' work, with its emphasis on the limitations of conventional ethics case narratives such as these (Chambers 1999). Traditional narratives, Chambers has shown, exhibit and suffer from, their status as "just-so" stories. In order to provide a focused, pertinent case illustration of the issue or issues at hand, they exhibit a post hoc staging of the case from an impersonal or omniscient standpoint. In this respect, they are overly, and artificially, neat.

Because they are in the third person, moreover, traditional case descriptions marginalize the internal experiences of the "actors" involved, presenting a unidimensional profile of each case participant. A person's character and its virtues, as we have seen, are revealed as much through inner states as by outwardly observable action or behavior of any kind—habits of mind, passing thoughts and feelings, deep, habituated attitudes framing initial response, temptations recognized and overcome, and so on. For this reason, inner monologue (or "self-talk") and responses known only to the subject, must be especially revealing when we try to understand the traits of character required by a virtue ethics approach such as the one adopted here. In the cases that follow, some of these inner responses, identified below in italics, are permitted to form part of the case narrative.

This suggests a further reason to eschew the method of traditional case narratives and to render the inner life of the clinician as participant in these exchanges. Only by doing so do we witness the inclinations that must be overcome in order to respond ethically. Traits such as forbearance, patience, and unselfing, for example, are associated with a rich and distinctive inner drama of contestation, persuasion, and maneuver. First impulses and natural inclinations are checked and curbed; "on balance" assessments are marshaled; such gentler states as benevolence and good sense are granted a chance to be felt and heard; the facts of the matter are subject to reassessment and reexamination and, sometimes, an overall reorientation of the whole case takes place. With the successful integration of those traits into one's character, these inner events become, to a greater or lesser degree, habitual; moreover, even when the achievement of forbearance, patience or unselfing are hard won, the effect, to the observer, will be seemingly swift and effortless. Despite their centrality to the moral life of the person, then, those experiences of inner struggle might well be completely absent from a third person narrative viewpoint. The virtuous clinician thinks before speaking and acting! And the empathic clinician who has mastered unselfing may give away little to an observer beyond the mien and body language of that empathy. Indeed, as empathy becomes a habit rather than a task, the clinician transitions and grows in virtue.

To re-create the inner states and responses of the clinician is not to diminish the extent to which the virtuous clinician is embedded in, and a product of, her interpersonal world. While her responses are informed by social exchange and empathic efforts to understand others, her access to that interpersonal world is still by way of her own distinctive and idiosyncratic perspective. It is useful, nonetheless, to approach case narratives so as to emphasize and highlight the internal perspective of the clinician. And ironically, even the narrative device of having the story told by only one protagonist offers opportunity to illustrate the leavening of a single viewpoint by those of others. In the case narratives that follow we see not narrative or hermeneutic certainty, but a subject continually receptive to the interpersonal context and other perspectives.

A fourth advantage associated with the nontraditional approach adopted in the case narratives making up this final chapter concerns the way it reveals the tensions and conflicts incumbent in the practitioners' role. Merely possessing virtues, as we have seen throughout this book, is often not enough without the metavirtue of *phronesis* that allows us to adapt to the particularities of practical situations. Clinical settings are filled with dilemmas, puzzles, and seeming contradictions, when the practitioner is tugged in incompatible directions and must choose which response, from a range, is the right and appropriate one. Including the practitioner's inner monologue in these case narratives allows us to observe some of this tension, conflict, and complexity, and its resolution. Narrating our cases from the viewpoint of the psychiatrist-actor reveals the subtlety of the virtue approach as well as the play of the virtues in the enactment of the professional psychiatric role.

Each of the cases that follow goes beyond the basic doctor–patient exchange of individual treatment that has been the mainstay of our case illustrations thus far. In contrast to the popular image of the psychiatrist as the lone practitioner in the office with an individual in distress, she is often embedded in a web of treatment-pertinent relationships with a panoply of actors. Cases 1–5 all show some added complexity arising with aspects of the practitioner's professional role: when there is more than one patient (Case 1); understood from within the broader perspective of the supervisory context (Case 2); when the goal and good of public safety must be added to that of healing (Case 3); concerning conflicts around professional duties and roles (Case 4); and finally, when the context includes the managed health care setting (Case 5).

This unconventional approach to ethics case writing, we emphasize, still yields cases that remain, finally, illustrative fictions. And although our hope is that they are revelatory fictions and not banal ones, like all case narratives, they are ambiguous and open to additional interpretation. Developing amalgamated cases in a way that renders them credible depictions of clinical reality while still serving the heuristic purpose of illustrating the theory of the preceding chapters proved unexpectedly difficult. As collaborators we wondered: How much, and which, aspects of inner monologue are sufficient to convey these inner states and stand as representative for a fuller stream of consciousness? Can a male clinician understand the subjectivity of a female clinician for the sake of portraying one? Should our analyses speculate on the character of other actors in the vignettes? Even striving for candor, can the clinician avoid face saving and flattering descriptions to the extent required for a realistic depiction?

The conventions for the following cases are: identifying a case number and title, a brief statement of context for the case, and the clinician's internal monologue set off in italics. An asterisk (*) between sections of dialogue suggests a transition to a later time.

Case 1:   Molecules and Marital Politics

Context: 14th session of couple therapy, but medication management involved

... I can't believe I'm thinking about suggesting this woman take an antidepressant—the citalopram ...

Rae rants and fidgets: "All Bill does when he comes home is flop down on the sofa in front of the TV and zone out ... I want to have a life with my husband ... I've suggested that we take a walk together, or plan some new things for the house, or go do something at the museum or whatever, and he just sort of goes along with what I'm saying and is agreeable but doesn't follow through. It's like he is sort of tolerating me rather than connecting with me ... "

"Look" Bill says. "I don't think it's unfair for me to unwind a little after a hard day's work and not have to take care of my wife's every need the moment I come through the door ... "

... here we go again ... dueling realities ... at what point do I interrupt this? ...

"Rae has been relentless in nagging me—I know she hates it when I say that, but its true ... I know I'm the bad communicator ... "

... we have the immoveable object meeting the irresistible force ... they have been cycling through this approach/avoidance dance for years ...

"You just don't get it ... what's the point of us being together if we're just roommates, and ones that don't talk either? I've tried being nice, I've tried being creative ... you just don't want to be with me ... " she says.

...perhaps I can introduce the issue of meds for Rae and put it into the context of a gender-role transaction they either can buy into, or not...

"Now hold on," he says, "we've had a lot of great times together, why just last weekend we went out with the Forts and you were happy and laughing...it seems like you're never satisfied...I think it's because you went off the citalopram...you've been bitchy ever since..."

"Here's my opening...for an alternate spin...And I can't resist...but let's hope the time is right..."

I interrupt: "Do you think that things are worse since going off the citalopram, Rae?"

"I'm just livid with him, it's just like he expects me to do all the adjusting...I have been more angry and irritable in the past few months..."

Me again: "Have you had depressive symptoms again?"

She never had DSM-IV major depression—just irritability and some depressed mood...I can see that the angrier she is, the more he pulls back, which of course makes her angrier...even in the best of times he's adrift in his football world...the irony is she is the one who has been more flexible and adaptive...he just pulls back from conflict and from her, always has, even in his prior relationships...does he have either the will or the capacity to be closer to her?

"...but why should I be the one who takes the pills to make me Miss Contentment? Why can't you give him some sort of 'sensitive male' pill?"

Now there's an idea. Talk about cultural differences, right here in one marriage!

I reply, "Unfortunately we haven't invented a sensitive male pill yet, so that's not much of an option. Do you really think that the citalopram makes you into a docile compliant female?"

That sounded pretty lame, but let's see how she responds....

"I think that's what he wants..."

"No I don't—I just don't want my ass chewed day in and day out..." Bill retorts.

(She continues, ignoring him) "...but it does make me feel better, and we do seem to do better when I'm on it, but it doesn't seem fair for him to get off scot free..."

Ah, fairness—I'm with her, but fairness is one of the toughest issues to settle... this could take forever....

"The question for me is whether you think going back on the citalopram is for you to be compliant with him, or whether you think it helps restore you to who you are..." I offer.

Maybe I should have said "and/or"... It can have both effects: is she able to see that? . . but this would sound like a real estate contract... and even more lame...

"I'd happily accept her restored AND compliant..." This is from Bill.

I suppress a wince. The guy does not get the picture that he is bungling his own case.

Rae doesn't suppress hers, and then directs a wry grimace at me.

She's looking for backup. What's the right metaphor?...

"Bill, you're shooting yourself in the foot again." I prompt.

"I know, but let's face it, she married a redneck."

This case offers what might be conventionally construed as a dilemma, in that the clinician must choose between medicating the wife into a compliant role, or taking on the project of remaking Bill, the self-professed redneck, into a sensitive postfeminist male. In this respect, the case highlights the question of how to honor the value of gender sensitivity. Bill's point of view is deeply antithetical to the clinician's. Yet the virtues of gender sensitivity, described earlier, require a response that is understanding and empathic; the practitioner must place himself imaginatively in Bill's place and try to see the world through his eyes. The adroit wording ("Bill, you're shooting yourself in the foot again") avoids any hint of disgust or rejection and, despite the bluster of his last remark, leads Bill toward a possible reassessment of his "redneck" ideology.

Treating a couple rather than an individual highlights the importance of emphasis on the unfolding of a process and dialogue. Instead of seeing this situation as one that must be settled by the clinician to his moral satisfaction, it is fed back to the couple for collaborative "deliberation." Most theoretical models of couple therapy portray this challenge in terms of the need for the therapist to possess "neutrality." He must be viewed as siding with neither partner; instead, the therapist is regarded by the couple as being on "both" of their sides, and as an advocate for both. Some of the internal monologue above reveals the therapist's struggle with maintaining such neutrality. ("Now there's an idea." "I suppress a wince.") Here is a situation that calls for self-knowledge, propriety, and unselfing. The awareness of his own bias regarding gender-role issues and sexism, also evident in his internal asides, will have required self-knowledge and a full understanding of his own gender identity and gender politics. Propriety and unselfing are evidenced in the inhibition of the therapist's judgmental wince. The clinician also requires *phronesis* here, the metavirtue that allows one to know how to respond in particular circumstances. This case illustrates a circumstance where neutrality must be maintained, because neutrality is necessary for the cooperation with and investment in each member of the couple.

Here, too, the practitioner exhibits realism. He assesses and deliberates about the relative immutability of Bill's character in comparison with the responsiveness of Rae to the antidepressant. Additional questions of "gender politics" remain to be negotiated among the three—and the therapist will no doubt find himself returning to these qualities of tact, unselfing, propriety, realism, *phronesis*, and gender sensitivity as he attempts to steer between the couples' differing ideas and values about gender roles while at the same time honoring their apparent shared goal of reconciling those ideas and values.

Case 2: Possible Predator

Context: ninth session of combined medication/psychotherapy treatment of a general hospital inpatient due for imminent discharge. [Dr. Jenner is a woman resident trainee, administratively supervised on the inpatient unit by Dr. Moore, and is supervised for psychotherapy treatment by Dr. Ritter.]

"…I should probably tell you that I have had thoughts about visiting your house…" he says, looking me straight in the eye.
It's the end of the session, of course. Should I be annoyed or afraid?
"Tell me more about what you mean."
Do I really want to know this?… this may end up being "TMI"—too much information… But you can't leave it there…

He returns to staring at the floor. "You know, I think about going to your house and watching you…(hesitating) it's a sexual type thing…I know it's inappropriate…" trailing off.

Let's see if he goes on…How much of this do I need to explore?…I'll definitely have some things to discuss in supervision . . .

"These temptations you've had…have you given in to them and actually gone to my house?"
I know I probably should have waited to ask this, but I had to know. This creep is beginning to scare me.
"No. Not yet. I mean I've resisted them. I need your help."
"Have you searched out my home address?" *I deadpan to hide my inner shudder.*
"….well, its 3408 Sycamore, Apt. 114…."
I suppress the second wave of shuddering. But he's looking at me in a new way now, as if he senses my unease…fear…and he's seems a little more confident!…
"Well, we should probably pick this up at the end of your next session. Same time next week?"
"That'll work," he says, leaving a little more briskly than usual.
This is freaking me out…I should probably ask Dr. Moore about this right away. They were planning to discharge this guy on Friday.

*

"Thanks for seeing me about Mr. Zeletsky. What I wanted to talk to you about so quickly is that in session yesterday he told me about his fantasies to 'look' in my house and that it was a 'sexual' thing. I understand you were going to discharge him, and I don't feel safe."
He's giving me his serious look. Good, I've got his attention at least.
"Dr. Jenner, let's slow down and think this through. What do we know about this guy? First, his diagnosis lies somewhere in the Asperger's-schizotypal netherworld. He's an odd sort, no friends to speak of, spends most of his time surfing the Web for porn, and drawing weird creatures of indeterminate gender. He's not a bad draftsman. His parents put up with him at home and are probably too aged to give him much trouble about his lifestyle. He's been

arrested a few times for peeping. Hasn't held a job for 5 years. He came to us after a serious suicide threat, though he hasn't ever made an attempt. He's never physically assaulted anyone as far as we know. He's perked up his mood with an antidepressant. I can understand your anxiety response, but what do you think we should do?"

The smug asshole.

"....I don't know, I just feel like I need more time to work more with him while he's in the hospital...talk to my supervisor...get a handle on this. I don't know if my creepy feelings are going to get in the way of working with him. I think he was picking up on my responses even today."

"You'll work it out." Moore says.

Easy for you to say. You're a 6'4" man.

*

"Are you ready for me?"

Dr. Ritter's always so busy.

"Of course—it's time for your supervision already?"

"Yes—and boy, do I have some stuff to tell you."

"I'm listening."

There's that rat like grin. Looks can be deceiving.

"Do you remember that inpatient I mentioned to you, with a history of suicidal ideation, depression, maybe Asperger's, and voyeurism?"

"Yes, but we really didn't discuss."

"I know, but in the last session he talked about wanting to come to my house and look in on me...he even said it was in a 'sexual' way. It was at the end of the session and so we didn't get to talk about it. But it freaked me out, and I'm wondering if I can work with someone who is scary to me. The thought of him lurking outside of my house is awful. I live by myself. But I don't know what to do. Just terminating with him is not a good answer; he could still end up at my house."

He's turned serious; he can see I'm freaked.

"I don't remember if he was dangerous or not. Has he committed crimes or assaulted anyone?"

"He has been arrested as a peeping Tom a few times over the years. As far as I know he hasn't done anything, but we are still early in the therapy and he's having these erotic feelings."

"Are you doing a psychodynamic-type treatment?"

"No, I didn't think he was a candidate for that at all. Mostly I'm working supportively with him and problem-solving his practical situations with him. I talked with Dr. Moore about it, and while I was scared about the session, I ended up kind of angry with him."

"Moore? Or the patient?"

"Dr. Moore. I thought his response was insensitive. The patient is a registered sex offender and Dr. Moore just sort of brushed off my concern. He just talked about how the patient has no history of dangerousness to others and told me I would work it out."

"But what about the patient—how did he seem about the matter? Casual? Embarrassed? Leering? And you haven't said much yet about his vulnerabilities."

Oh yeah. The patient.

"The patient was kinda uncomfortable about the whole thing, from what I observed, but testing, too. Watching his effect on me .... "

This says something right there about this patient's dynamics—I'll need to bring this up again later with Ritter.

"I can understand how you'd be freaked out by this sort of thing. What's the next step?"

"I think I need to talk to Dr. Moore about the discharge plan for Friday. Maybe he would be more negotiable if I spoke to him in more detail."

Puh-leeze, I'm not a kid—I can take this up with Moore.

"That's okay—I appreciate it but you've given me some perspective and I can speak to Moore on my own."

"Is anyone supervising your therapy with this patient?"

"No, not really. I only have two supervisors, and they only want to hear one, or at most two, cases."

"Well, we could set aside Mrs. Smith as she is pretty stable, and perhaps talk more about this patient in detail. Maybe you should present him to me again, from the top, and refresh my memory."

One aspect that distinguishes this case is the role of particular virtues in understanding hierarchical professional relationships. Dr. Jenner is a resident trainee. Dr. Moore is responsible for her supervision on the inpatient unit and Dr. Ritter for the psychotherapy treatment she undertakes with patients. A power differential exists between Dr. Jenner and the two faculty psychiatrists. She confides in Dr. Ritter, not just in the particulars of the clinical case, but also about the strained situation with Dr. Moore. We can see from the inner monologue that Dr. Jenner likes or respects Ritter more than Moore, at least during the stretch of time within which this scenario takes place. With Jenner's recounting, Ritter listens carefully but (presumably) respectfully and temperately, saying nothing about the relationship with Moore in this vignette. Indeed, Dr. Ritter redirects her to patient concerns. Later Dr. Jenner comes to her own conclusions about going back and revisiting the case with Dr. Moore, exhibiting her own recognition that this is a perspective she should integrate to fully understand how to respond in this case. Moreover, she realizes she should address the residual conflict with Dr. Moore herself.

Earlier in the case, we see Dr. Jenner's frustration and annoyance with Dr. Moore, but she discreetly, and perhaps patiently, keeps her "smug asshole" assessment (and affect) to herself. Dr. Jenner's frustration with Moore requires her to draw upon propriety as she assimilates some perspective through time, discussion with Ritter, and reflection. Impulsively blurting out her annoyance with Moore would accomplish nothing.

Early in this case, Dr. Jenner realizes with an inner, controlled, shudder that Mr. Zeletsky has thought about, and perhaps already, stalked her. In psychoanalytic parlance this "countertransference" reaction, however understandable, raises the question of Dr. Jenner's ability to work effectively with the patient. Her frankness with her supervisors about this fact demonstrates the embodiment of self-effacement and truthfulness in practice. Dr. Jenner confesses her vulnerability in this case and effectively seeks counsel with supervisors.

In Chapter 5 we discussed the meaning of empathy and compassion as related virtues, emphasizing the practiced cultivation of an understanding of and concern for patients. As a resident trainee, Dr Jenner is not only learning the facts of psychiatry but also the dispositions and comportment of the clinician. With such trainees the cultivation and habituation of empathy and compassion often occur within the context of psychotherapy supervision and training, where the resident is directed toward using her imagination to recognize the vulnerability underneath the angry, provocative, seductive, or

arrogant veneer of the patient. Through the widening of her emotional perception of people beyond the immediate reflexive response to provocation,
and the integration of the provocation into a more holistic understanding of
the patient's vulnerabilities, "defenses," and assets, the clinician cultivates the
empathy she will require for effective practice. We see a gentle push toward
cultivating a more mature or encompassing empathy through the remark by
supervisor Ritter regarding patient Zeletsky's vulnerabilities, with Jenner's
subsequent "Oh yeah, the patient" response, revealing her own reawakened
awareness.

Only *phronesis*, with its power to adjudicate among the different possible responses she might envision, can guide Dr Jenner as to which virtues are apt in the situation of a vulnerable patient, driven to behavior he
recognizes as wrongful, who reluctantly confesses desires or thoughts that
he likely realizes will be upsetting to the very person he seeks help from.
Might we say Dr. Jenner is being inauthentic in hiding her true feelings
about the patient? Dr. Jenner intuits that sharing her fearful response with
the patient at that moment will likely prevent the patient from being open
with her. Indeed, had she done so, the patient would likely have hidden his
feelings, as he has from others, and compounded his isolation and alien-
ation. Such emotional closing-off could even aggravate the obsessive symptoms. The patient's confidence in Jenner's ability to help would likely have
been undermined, moreover. Were it perceived, Dr. Jenner's shudder would
undermine her relationship with the patient, accomplishing nothing. In this
context, the virtues of authenticity or "genuineness" mean the clinician keeps
her focus and discipline directed toward the patient's interests, rather than
her transient personal comfort. And achieving self-control—or unselfing—in
this moment demonstrates Dr Jenner's genuine and benevolent concern with
Mr. Zeletsky's needs and interests.

Case 3:   Death Threats

*Context: Day 8 of an inpatient stay in a general-hospital psychiatric
unit for a patient (Preminger) who was voluntarily hospitalized for
a delusional psychosis involving death threats to his fellow workers
in the Post Office. The unit chief and the treating psychiatrist are
discussing discharge in an office.*

"One issue with his discharge is his work disposition. The post office has already told him they don't want him back at their location."

"They can't just fire him because he's ill ... "

"They're not talking about firing him, they're talking about transferring him to another facility where he can have a "fresh start" and not have everyone in the shop afraid of him. The patient has actually been talking with his postmaster at the old location and has settled on the new location. The questions are whether he is ready for discharge and what we should do about warning his soon-to-be former coworkers. How do you think Preminger is doing?

"Well, in terms of his psychotic symptoms, the voices are mostly gone, but I'm not so confident about the resolution of his paranoid delusions about the coworkers. He is, I think, spontaneously questioning the reality of his delusions, and certainly they're not as compelling as they were before, but his insight into his illness is still pretty shaky."

"What makes you say that?"

"Little things. He still wants to read his *Soldier of Fortune* magazines and he's still drawing battle scenes in art therapy. He still is pretty guarded with everyone. He still has an occasional rant about the post office out in the open area with the other patients. I'm not so sure all of his complaints are delusional though."

"Let's interview him together this afternoon and decide from that."

*

"Mr. Preminger, I had mentioned to you this morning that Dr. Bates and I would be coming by this afternoon to talk to you about your discharge. Have a seat—can we get you some water or juice?"

"No thanks."

"Tell us how you've been doing over your hospital stay."

He's frowning and staring at the floor ... I look at Bates, wondering what he makes of these responses.

"Well, since I got back on my medicine, the voices have gone away, and my sleep is better. ... When do I get to go home?"

"We're not sure yet, but you should probably also tell us about the nanobots."

He really got going about the nanobots when he came in.

"Do you know about them?"

He's looking at Bates, who is impassive. *What can Bates be making of this?*

"Just from what your chart described when you came in, and what Dr. Williams has told me."

"How much do you want me to say?"

He looks at me like a kid asking permission, as if he wants to keep going ... is eager to tell.

"Tell us what you think is important for us to know."

"....when I came in I was sure that Karen and Jack were leading the campaign to put nanobots into my coffee and cigarettes ... you know they are heat-resistant, like Teflon ... and that the nanobots were slowly killing me because I was leading the Rebellion . . . people on the Rebellion web page were encouraging me to go to the police, but you know they don't believe me .... . but now it seems kind of dumb, like my imagination, especially since the voices have gone away and quit giving orders to retaliate ... "

He trails off—does that mean that he's said it all, or is having doubts now, about what he's revealed...getting frightened, frightening himself again?

"Do you think you're still in danger?"

"Well, not really. You and the nurses have been telling me this is part of my illness and the medicine seems to have made my worries about the Rebellion and nanobot attacks less important ... "

"How do the people at the post office feel about you?"

"I don't know ... you've told me that some of the employees are afraid of me and don't want me back ... the postmaster is going to transfer me ... "

"Do you think that's a good idea?"

Oops, leading the patient.

"I guess, but I won't get to see Harriet much anymore, and she was about the only person at work I could talk to ... are you going to commit me?"

Think fast.

"Well, you know that when you came in you were threatening to kill Jack and Karen, and we had considered committing you then, but you agreed to sign in for treatment, and we didn't have to. You know we have to assure your safety, and be sure that you are not dangerous to other people. Do you think you will be safe?"

"I still don't much like Jack and Karen, but wanting to kill them seems dumb. I'll be OK, unless the voices tell me to stop taking my medication."

"What can you do to prevent that?"

"By taking my medicine, keeping my appointments with you, and telling you about the first sign of voices."

A little on the rote side. Will he follow through?

"You might think about people at home and around that you might be able to get help from for these things. Dr. Bates and I were wondering if we should warn Karen and Jack and maybe others about you, in case your worries about the nanobots and the voices come back. What do you think?"

"I don't know. You're the doctors. Do you think the voices will come back?"

"Definitely, if you don't take your medicine. Dr. Bates and I will think about this some more and come back to discuss with you."

This case offers the opportunity to consider the relationship of virtues to professional duties and standards. Moreover, the case involves complex clinical judgments with moral as well as professional significance (such as the questions of involuntarily secluding the patient as well as warning the possible victims). These are not merely complex judgments, moreover. They are high-stakes ones—involving the patient's and others' safety and security.

The practitioner's concern here is not just for the patient, but for coworkers or unidentified others who may be at risk. This concern, so common in clinical practice, is an expression of the virtue of benevolence, which makes up part of the tacit and often overlooked background of the virtuous character in any professional role. Other virtues present here are the self-knowledge and humility discussed in Chapter 5. Unseasoned practitioners without these virtues will be tempted to respond to the high-stakes ambiguities of psychiatric practice with self-reassuring expressions of certitude about matters that remain quite uncertain. The approach of both doctors here reveals doubt and humility, appropriate virtues in the face of this kind of common, but always demanding, situation. The protagonist, Dr. Williams, reveals his doubt through his inner monologue at several steps in the interview.

Humility not tempered by fortitude and perseverance, however, will likely result in passivity and inaction, and a temptation for many clinicians would be to defer discharge and prolong the hospital stay. Although tempting, this decision may not benefit the patient, but merely delay or dodge the heavy responsibility of discharging him. The emotional burden of worry about the unpredictable behavior of dangerous patients is one of the greatest challenges in psychiatric practice. To reduce or avoid that worry, the practitioner is inclined to disregard the patient's interests and the realities of the case. Self-knowledge, to recognize this temptation; realism, to assess the risks and facts; fortitude and perseverance, to avoid inertia in the face of uncertainty, are all required in such circumstances. And so too is *phronesis*, in judging when to tolerate uncertainty over dangerous patients, and how to reduce uncertainty without shirking basic obligations to the patient's well-being.

Virtues more evident in this case vignette are suggested by the forthright manner in which the clinicians engage Mr. Preminger. They are frank about their social-psychiatric obligations to at least consider the possibility of warning potential victims and involve Preminger directly in their deliberations.

Case 4: The Gatekeeper (adapted from Sadler 1986)

Context: An interview room in an emergency psychiatry service of a large, urban county hospital. The Stevens parents have arranged for a court-ordered evaluation for their 25-year-old schizophrenic son, Robert, because of threatening them at knifepoint yesterday evening. The couple is present with the son for the evaluation conducted by Dr. Gutierrez. The interview here is picked up at midpoint.

"Robert, how about having a seat and letting us complete the interview … right there is fine."

How many times now have I asked him to sit down? He's so agitated, and the question is when to raise the question of medicating him—now, or later.

"He's just this way at home, isn't he Mark? He won't sit and won't listen …" this is his mother, Rachel. Husband Mark sits quietly, nodding in agreement, his face impassive and distant.

Mark's ready to get out of here, maybe more than Robert …

"He hasn't been taking his medicine at all in the past three months..." Rachel continues.

"That's a lie!" Robert interrupts, "You're always lying to them to get them to lock me up."

I impulsively jump in: "And who is the 'them' who are lying to you, Robert?"

"The conspiracy. You all are in it. I can tell from the smell." Robert says suspiciously.

"What smell?" *I wonder about idiosyncratic thinking or the window into a delusional system.*

"The dry cleaning smell on your clothes. That's the way you know who is on the side of the conspiracy."

Hypothesis confirmed.

(Rachel, interrupting and turning to Dr. Gutierrez, voice raised) "You're not going to let him carry on about this nonsense again are you? We've been over this a million times! He needs to be in the hospital to get back on his medicines. He won't take them at home. This is the ninth time we've had to do this in the past 5 years. Why don't you take the family seriously? You can see that the boarding home couldn't handle him. You all are just trying to save money."

Uh oh. Mom's escalating, Dad's hapless, and Robert is just now letting down his guard, opening up some firmer evidence of psychosis...

"They didn't kick me out, I left because they were working for the Conspiracy." Robert interjects.

What this family needs is some psychoeducation sessions... I wonder why they've never been offered...

A knock on the door, and the unit administrator says "Dr. Gutierrez, you have a phone call."

Saved by the bell, but I have to face the music again shortly!

*

(Dr. Gutierrez exits and returns a few minutes later after the call.)

*

(To the family)

"Y'all, what I have is this. Robert left the boarding house because he believes they are in cahoots with the Conspiracy, though the rest of us believe this is a symptom of his illness. Mr. and Mrs. Stevens, you think Robert threatened you at knifepoint at the dinner table last night and Robert says he was 'just making a point with the [dinner] knife in my hand.' Everyone agrees, I think, that he has never harmed anyone and just gets angry and threatening. Robert says he is willing to take his medicine as an outpatient, though (turning to Robert) you know you often don't follow through. (Turning to parents) My exam indicates that Robert has not changed much or "deteriorated" as we say, enough for us to justify putting him in the hospital involuntarily. He doesn't meet the commitment criteria. He refuses to go in voluntarily.

I can "throw the parents a bone" and test Robert's willingness to take medicine by getting him started here… and maybe they won't threaten to sue me.

"I'm afraid all I can do is refill his prescription here, and make arrangements for a quick clinic visit. I should ask Robert to take a dose of his medicine here in the ER before he is discharged. Robert, would you be willing to do this?"

Please say yes Robert.

Rachel (interrupting) "No!" Mark shakes his head disgustedly.

Robert (simultaneously) "OK."

Sometimes you just can't win.

"Dr. Gutierrez, you're supposed to help us, and you haven't done anything. If something happens we're going to call our attorney. Mark, let's wait outside." They storm out of the room and head for the waiting room.

"Robert, the nurse, Mrs. Smith, will be in shortly to give you your medicine."

Robert: "Can I have a cigarette now?"

In Chapter 6, we discussed conflicts imposed on practitioners when they are called upon to undertake seemingly incompatible roles. In the emergency room setting Dr Gutierrez is required to act as a gatekeeper, placing the interests of public safety as implied legal duties governing involuntary treatment ahead of many fiduciary responsibilities to the patient before him. This is not a simple task: to even determine where Robert's case lies in relation to those rules, he must also establish enough rapport with the patient to obtain grounds for his clinical judgment that Robert's disorder, anger, and distress will be unlikely to end in violence. To achieve this he must preserve apparent neutrality, not seeming to favor Rachel's perspective over Robert's own. The whole family is important to the evaluation and disposition, and Dr. Gutierrez tries to maintain credibility with parents and patient. He must also seize the opportunity to explore Robert's remarks about the conspiracy, since this will establish good evidence for Robert's chronically psychotic state, which the case vignette implies has been suppressed or "guarded" by Robert in the earlier parts of the interview. Overall, though, these "therapeutic" interview techniques must in this context be placed in the service not of healing but of reaching an informed judgment as to the patient's state of mind in relation to legal definitions, and providing a reasonable enough clinical relationship with all parties to facilitate follow-though into the next level of care.

Even this much analysis does not do justice to the complexity of Dr. Gutierrez' case. Note we mentioned "implied" legal duties. What involuntary treatment laws provide in many jurisdictions is "permission" for psychiatrists to involuntary seclude or treat dangerous patients, but in the law "permission" is not the same as "obligation" or "duty." Whether or not to commit Robert is a medical decision that is authorized by the State, but doesn't compel Dr. Gutierrez to act in any direct way other than secure a medically defensible treatment plan or intervention. What makes Dr. Gutierrez so skittish? The ever-looming specter of malpractice suits haunts psychiatrists in emergency settings, where so often adequate treatment options are few and expectations to deliver miracles are high. Hence the legal permission to commit may not be an obligation, but *feels* like one to the clinician in the emergency department. Indeed, many less-virtuous clinicians might pursue the route of least resistance and simply go ahead and commit Robert to "cover my (the doctor's) ass." Dr. Gutierrez draws upon his perseverance, courage, and integrity when he attempts to address multiple needs: to not misuse his commitment privilege, to aid the parents *and* Robert, to apply the law fairly, to make practical, effective use of limited resources, and of course, not get sued.

In some instances, we pointed out earlier, role conflicts such as these may be so extreme as to leave the practitioner no choice but to relinquish one or the other role. He cannot wear both hats. Such dual, even multiple, roles seem an inevitable part of the practice setting and, as we saw, the practitioner may avoid moral hazard when the ends or goals of each role—here, public safety and treatment—are themselves morally justified and acceptable to him, and when the virtue of integrity is cultivated. Nonetheless, the practitioner will likely suffer from the attempt to fulfill the role of therapist alongside that of gatekeeper, as Dr. Gutierrez clearly does in this case. The priorities may be clear enough and agreed upon. The doctor is legally and morally bound to prevent harm to other people before, or instead of, attending to the patient's symptoms. And similarly, when the patient's danger of self-harm meets a certain, legally defined and clinically interpreted threshold, responding to that danger must take precedence. (See Sadler 1986.) But the unmet impulse to treat a patient as unquestionably troubled and disordered as Robert will bring discomfort and chagrin to the practitioner even as he recognizes and responds to these imperatives.

And when the priorities are clear, the facts of the matter may yet remain uncertain. As this case indicates, the family system, including an apparently enmeshed mother and disengaged father, must affect and will likely need to frame any accurate understanding of Robert's symptoms. Dr Gutierrez's determination that Robert does not qualify as an involuntary patient is an assessment made in light of the behavior of all three family members.

As a determination about a complex disorder made on the basis of a cursory interview in the rushed emergency room setting, it should also be added, Dr. Gutierrez's assessment will need *phronesis*. His request that Robert take the first dose of medicine there and then indicates evidence of just such a virtue. Dr. Gutierrez' instruction to take medicine before discharge from the ER tests Robert's willingness to take medicine as an outpatient (at least for now), permits an opportunity to observe Robert for adverse reactions that may contribute to his ambivalence about taking medications, and indicates to the parents that the physician is at least taking their concerns into some degree of consideration. Phronetic clinical work that packs multiple objectives into a few interventions makes for elegant, if far-from-perfect, care.

Case 5: Paying for Psychotherapy

Context: Telephone screening interview of a woman seeking help for marital problems.

"Is this Mrs. Wright? This is Dr. Washington returning your call. Is this a convenient place and time for you to talk?"
"Yes, but let me pick it up in another room."

"OK."

"I'm back. Thanks for returning my call so promptly. I'm not sure where to start."

"You should tell me a little about what sort of problems you've been having, to see if I'm the right doctor for you. Also, I understand you are covered by the HealthMore plan from your employer, and one of the things HealthMore requires for mental health care is that I have to 'pre-certify' you so that they will pay for your initial evaluation visit."

"That's what I heard. I think the problem has to do with my marriage. Dick has been working longer and longer hours, comes home exhausted and tense—just wants to flop down on the sofa and watch TV. He gets annoyed if I interrupt him and often it turns into a shouting match. This has been going on for months. It's gotten to the point that I avoid him, and I've thought about divorce or even thinking life is not worth living."

"What other ways has the relationship affected you personally?"

"I've had trouble sleeping, keeping my mind on things at work. I come home at 3:30 and just want to sleep—nothing seems much fun or interesting. I think I might have clinical depression."

This sounds rather rote. What does she really want? Can we get some sort of corroboration here? Does the spouse even know about this?

"Do you think your husband would be willing to come in also?"

"Yes, he agrees that we should work together on this. He thinks we need marital counseling. His father was a pastor and saw how his father's work could help married people."

Has she found an acceptable presenting symptom that may be concealing other problems?

"Is there anything else going on that I must know right now? General health problems?"

"No. You should have a referral form from my regular doctor, Dr. Cook."

"I do, and it answers the other questions I might have in terms of presenting this to the HealthMore people. Let me call them and set up the precertification, and someone from our office will call you back to set up an appointment."

*

[Conclusion of the precertification call, where the case information above was presented to the precertification reviewer]

"Dr. Washington, you understand while I'm certifying this evaluation appointment, the HealthMore contract from this particular employer excludes reimbursement for marital psychotherapy—you'll need to bill this out as Mrs. Wright's DSM or ICD diagnosis. You'll then need to present a treatment plan for approval."

I knew this was going to happen. Why can't these people see how mood disorders and marital relationships are interrelated?

*

"I thought you would want to know that your HealthMore contract doesn't pay for marital therapy, so I would have to bill your care to them as an individual patient."

"Dr. Washington, that's awful…Dick will be angry about this……Would it be possible for you to see both of us and bill it out just under my name?"

She may not realize she's asking me to defraud her insurance company, but this is the sort of thing that discourages people like her from getting care at all.

While the preceding cases suggest other sample moments of "quick-thinking" demands, this one involving managed care is particularly acute—a fleeting moment in a telephone conversation. This kind of morally problematic fleeting moment, while by no means confined to psychiatry, is one that illustrates the pervasive every day demands on the role constituted virtues for psychiatric practitioners. Dr. Washington feels an obligation to serve the interests of his patient(s). He also wants to be paid. He presumably does not want to be paid through intentional or accidental defrauding of Mrs. Wright's insurance company.

This situation calls for several virtues, the most obvious of which is the ability to think quickly—at least in the first instance of this all-too-common problem. Only virtues that are deeply habituated in the character will permit the ready responses Dr Washington exhibits here, there is no time for reflection in a brief, telephone exchange. Here are honesty and integrity as well as empathy—honesty and integrity to see, and resist, the temptation offered by patient's suggestion that he cheat on the billing; empathy, to recognize that his patient is too distraught to be aware of, or care about, the implications of her proposal. The virtues of moral leadership required for the responsible attitude toward resource allocation referred to as stewardship (discussed in Chapters 3 and 5) are also evident in this brief vignette. Dr. Washington does not shirk from participation in efforts to manage and deliver health care resources and costs. He shows the traits necessary for the role imposed on those practicing within today's managed care delivery systems.

One of the central challenges of those systems, we saw earlier, is integrating stewardship responsibilities with other, more traditional and fiduciary ones and their corresponding virtues: fidelity (to the patient) and integrity (in preserving quality care), most notably. Such is the case with Dr. Washington's situation here. The apparent conflicts between "fiduciary" and "stewardship" virtues allow us to consider how some virtues can balance or regulate other ones.

In addition, the situation requires practical wisdom or *phronesis*. Dr. Washington must know how to navigate this particular company or employer contract for mental health services. The company may not pay for couple treatment for marital problems, for instance, but would fund couple treatment as a component treatment for one member of the couple who suffered depression. This could be explored with a phone call to the company. A delicate and nuanced propriety in dealing with Mrs. Wright is also indicated. Dr. Washington must choose his response carefully to avoid sounding dismissive of her question, or accusatory, through saying or implying that her request is fraudulent. He must convey concern and caring (fidelity, benevolence, genuineness) toward her while attending to his legitimate desire to be paid for his services. He can suggest to her now that he can "explore this possibility" with the insurance company and return to her with their decision. He will be required to contact the insurance company anyway for the precertification procedure, which will provide time for him to explore the billing codes. He can, however, go ahead and offer her an appointment time as a reassurance. If he can work out the reimbursement with HealthMore, fine, if not, he'll have to return to Mrs. Wright with alternatives, including treating her individually (less than ideal) or referring her to another clinician off-plan (because Dr. Washington may be contractually obligated to be paid only through HealthMore's management)—also less than ideal. A short telephone conversation can lead to an intensive phronetic workout!

When Dr. Washington does return with the decision, we would expect the prevailing virtue called for here would be trustworthiness and integrity regarding the billing issues, and empathy and benevolence toward Mrs. Wright.

8 Conclusion

Our emphasis throughout this book has been on the kind of character that seems best suited to the psychiatrist caring for those with severe mental disorders, and ways a virtue-focused approach enables us to acknowledge the distinctive ethical demands upon that practitioner. We have pointed out that the primary focus of these ideas will be the educational setting where trainees are being exposed to the ideals of the profession and taught their craft. Because of this emphasis on training, we want to close with a brief discussion of whether, and how, virtue can be taught, and with our prescriptive conclusion: along with training in clinical skills, those entering psychiatry must be taught to cultivate the added virtues and enhanced virtue called for by the professional role they are to undertake.

There are actually three questions that have been asked about teaching virtues in this kind of professional context, not two. The first is whether virtue *should* be taught: whether this kind of values and character training is appropriate. The second, raised earlier in this book, is whether virtue *can* be taught. And the third, also touched on earlier, is *how* it might be taught.

The first question is central to our efforts here. Our argument for the necessity of cultivating certain character virtues called for by the psychiatry setting has direct implications for the training of fledgling practitioners. Virtues, we conclude, *can* and *should* be taught.

This first question is not uncontroversial. Moral education is necessary for children and youth, of course—this is universally agreed upon. But some have resisted the teaching of virtue to adults acquiring professional training, emphasizing a contrast between moral qualities and value-neutral skills. The latter may safely be taught because they are value neutral, it is argued, but it would be inappropriate to teach virtues, because they are not.

This is a position with which we disagree. For effective and ethical practice in psychiatry, we hope to have demonstrated in the previous pages, virtues must be cultivated in trainee psychiatrists. Moreover, the very category of skills and traits that are entirely value neutral is a problematic one on several grounds. Writing of medical humanities training, for instance, Loretta Kopelman has demonstrated that values are inescapable, influencing every aspect of such a curriculum. It is impossible to analyze, explain, justify, criticize, or teach from an entirely neutral, or value-free, perspective. Rather than misguidedly attempting to avoid the values that underlie their curricula, Kopelman believes instructors should try to identify, explain, and justify them. (See Kopelman 1999: 1309.)

Especially when we recognize the nature of professional role morality, the distinction between capabilities that are virtues and those that are skills cannot be maintained, and the unsustainability of the claim that character training is *inappropriate* becomes doubly clear. Within role morality, the goals and goods of the practice—mental health and healing, in psychiatry—determine the whole ethical nature of the enterprise. Psychiatrists must achieve a successful alliance with the patient *because that relationship is necessary for healing, and healing is the regulative ideal of practice.* And as a precondition for effecting that alliance, being able to feel and communicate empathy must be construed as a valued virtue, not a value-neutral skill.

The question of whether virtue *can* be taught was one first raised by Socrates in the *Protagoras* on observing that there were no expert teachers of virtue. As we have noted before, Aristotle's emphasis on the way virtues can be cultivated through habituation is a response to that concern.

Part of the difficulty of supposing that virtues could not be taught seems to rest on a mistaken assumption—that virtues are unitary qualities. Yet, as we have demonstrated throughout this book, and as Aristotle's analysis makes very clear, they are far from that. Rather, virtues are a heterogeneous collection of states and traits, both when they are understood collectively and, as we have seen, when they are subject to individual examination. Many of these states and traits, moreover—attention, sensitivity, and efforts of imagination—are elements in any number of everyday, informal and formal learning, and central to much if not all education. So of the key subcapabilities underlying the cultivation of ·virtues some, at least, are qualities that are known to be responsive to training and practice.

Because it has been recognized that in adults subcapabilities such as sensitivity can be cultivated through training, such traits have been the focus of considerable recent attention within the domain of moral education. Moral reasoning skills, too, can be taught, it has been demonstrated (Rajczi 2003). That said, the preconditions for this adult learning, important recent work also suggests, include moral education during childhood and youth. What Martin Hoffman has called the "induction" of morally sensitive responses by parents to reinforce children's natural prosocial and sympathetic tendencies, seem to be essential building blocks here (Hoffman 2000). And perhaps only in an adult character prepared by such socialization, this suggests, can moral reasoning skills be taught.

As we noted at the outset, this early moral education, although important, is taken as a given throughout our discussion. Our psychiatry trainees, we assume, are young adults whose early education has equipped them with the normal capacity for moral responsiveness. With such people, research suggests, enhanced moral sensitivity, additional virtues, and greater virtue can be achieved.

Empathy is a paradigm example that has recently captured the interest and research of social psychologists, as well as nursing and medical educators (Authier 1986; Bennett 1995; Davis 1994; Henderson 2001; Irving and Dickson 2004; Larson and Yao 2005; Matthews et al. 1993; Zoppi and Epstein 2002). Several forms of pedagogy have been shown effective here (Karr 1994; Larson and Yao 2005). These include discussion of moral dilemmas and case materials in a classroom or group setting; cooperation-seeking games, role play and other simulation exercises, communication skill training, and journal keeping (Charon 2001; Rajczi 2003). Simulating the experiences of others these ways, as Robert Gordon has explained, allows us to extend to others "the modes of attribution, explanation, and prediction that otherwise would be applicable only in our own case" (Gordon 1995: 730).

In addition, examples and exemplars offer learners a concrete personification to guide their practice. Such role models may be real or imagined, actual or fictional. Whether through immediate contact or literary or cinematographic depictions, it is widely supposed that the learner will adopt and internalize the virtues so observed in respected and admired exemplars

(Larson and Yao 2005). And the importance of this sort of learning has long been recognized in the apprenticeship, practice-based model of medical education, it should be added.

Some of the pedagogical approaches outlined above are directed toward the particular subcapabilities making up virtues, others have been employed to cultivate the desired traits in their entirety—empathy, and other empathic emotions, in particular. Now included in a range of settings, efforts at "empathy training" are often designed to harness and enhance the imagination—again, through simulation, role play, exposure to literary and cinematographic works, journal keeping, and other forms of self-discovery and self-monitoring (Charon 2001; Deigh 1995; Gordon 1998; Ickes 1997; Shapiro et al. 2004; Vetlesen 1994).

In view of our earlier emphasis on the part played by empathic responses in practice, combined with the status of empathy as an unruly virtue, these techniques for instilling, strengthening, and augmenting empathy and related empathic emotions are especially important to our discussion. Because they are primarily affective, several of the practitioner's virtues identified in the preceding pages cannot be cultivated through direct approaches to training. Cultivating unruly virtues, of which empathy is one, depends on a different kind of training, as we have seen: the tendency to respond with empathy must be induced through practices that are less direct. And the above techniques suggest how this indirect learning can take place—through practice, by acquiring habits of mind such as imaginatively placing ourselves in the situation of the other person, and engaging in allied forms of simulation, for example. The role of imaginative capabilities in these exercises, it seems agreed, is central, and locates this discussion within Iris Murdoch's insightful analyses of the ingredients of moral learning. Murdoch speaks of a moral sense of "seeing" that results from "moral imagination and moral effort" (Murdoch 1967: 34).

In conclusion then, the role-generated virtues of psychiatric practice can be taught—or at least enhanced, deepened, and augmented. This will likely require that natural, affective, and social tendencies have been appropriately shaped during childhood. So trainees will almost certainly possess differing aptitudes for such learning, based on variability in their possession of those tendencies, as well as on the way such early moral education has been conducted.[1] Nonetheless, such training can, and should, be undertaken.

[1] See Davis (1983).

Some of the implications of this conclusion for residency training will be immediately obvious. (Although they are beyond the focus of the present work, so are the implications for evaluating applicants for such training. Moreover, the questions of whether virtues can be taught and their part in the selection of such candidates are seemingly interconnected. How easily and effectively virtues can be taught employing the kinds of pedagogy described above, will likely influence the weight placed on the characters and capacity for cultivating these professional virtues among applicants for psychiatry training.) An ethical approach that focuses on the character of the practitioner is a necessary and important ingredient in training for psychiatry. And the practical import of this conclusion is that skills and attitudes training must include the cultivation of greater moral responsiveness and enhanced virtue in residents, using pedagogies such as those outlined above. To ensure that the professional goals and goods of medicine are properly upheld and honored within psychiatric practice, we believe the practitioner should cultivate a virtuous character.

References

Agich, G. J. 1980. Professionalism and ethics in health care. *Journal of Medicine and Philosophy* 5 (3):186–99.

Alarcon, R. D. 2000. Culture and ethics of managed care in the United States. In *Ethics, culture & psychiatry: International perspectives*, ed. A. Okasha, J. Aboleda-Florez, and N. Sartorius, 83–102. Washington DC: American Psychiatric Association Press.

Alderson, P. 1991. Abstract bioethics ignores human emotions. *Bulletin of Medical Ethics* 168:13–21.

American Medical Association. 2000. *Principles of medical ethics*. Washington, DC: American Medical Press.

American Medical Association. 2000. *Current opinions and annotations 2000–2001 edition*. Washington, DC: American Medical Press: xiv.

American Psychiatric Association (APA). 2001. *The principles of medical ethics: With annotations especially applicable to psychiatry*. Washington, DC: American Psychiatric Association.

Appelbaum, P. 1997. A theory of ethics for forensic psychiatry. *Journal of the American Academy of Psychiatry and Law* 25:233–47.

Appelbaum, P., and L. Jorgenson. 1991. Psychotherapist-patient sexual contact after termination: An analysis and a proposal. *American Journal of Psychiatry* 148:1466.

Aristotle. 1985. *Nichomachean ethics*, trans. T. Irwin. Indianapolis: Hackett.

Aronowitz, R. 1998. *Making sense of illness: Science, society and disease*. Cambridge: Cambridge University Press.

Arpaly, N. 2003. *Unprincipled virtue: An inquiry into moral agency.* New York: Oxford University Press.

Ashton, H. 1991. Psychotropic-drug prescribing for women. *British Journal of Psychiatry* 158 (Suppl. 10):30–5.

Atkins, D., ed. 1998. *Looking queer: Body image and identity in lesbian, bisexual, gay and transgender communities.* New York: Haworth Press.

Authier, J. 1986. Showing warmth and empathy. In *A Handbook of Communication Skills,* ed. O. Hargie, 441–65. London: Croom Helm.

Baier, A. 1985. What do women want in a moral theory? *Nous* 19:53–63.

Baier, A. 1992. Trusting people. *Philosophical Perspectives.* 6:137–53.

Baier, A. 1995. *Postures of the mind: Essays on mind and morals.* Minneapolis: University of Minnesota Press.

Barham, P., and R. Hayward. 1991. *From the mental patient to the person.* London: Routledge.

Barham, P., and R. Hayward. 1995. *Relocating madness.* London: Free Association Books.

Barham, P. 1997. *Closing the asylum: The mental patient in modern society.* London: Penguin Books.

Barham, P., and R. Hayward. 1998. In sickness and in health: Dilemmas of the person with severe mental illness. *Psychiatry* 61:163–70.

Barker, P., Campbell, P., and B. Davidson, eds. 1999. *From the ashes of experience, reflections on madness, survival, growth.* London: Macmillan.

Baum, D. 2004. The price of valor. *The New Yorker,* 12 and 19 July, 44–52.

Bayer, R. 1981. *Homosexuality and American psychiatry: The politics of diagnosis.* New York: Basic Books.

Beauchamp, T. 1995. Principlism and its alleged competitors. *Journal of the Kennedy Institute of Ethics* 5:181–98.

Beauchamp, T. 1999. The philosophical basis of psychiatric ethics. In *Psychiatric Ethics, third edition,* ed. S. Bloch, P. Chodoff, and S. Green, 25–48. Oxford: Oxford University Press.

Beauchamp, T., and J. Childress. 2001. *Principles of biomedical ethics, fifth edition.* New York: Oxford University Press.

Bem, S. L. 1995. Dismantling gender polarization and compulsory heterosexuality. *Journal of Sex Research* 32:329–334.

Benatar, S. R. 1987. The changing doctor-patient relationship and the new medical ethics. *South African Journal of Continuing Medical Education* 5, April:27–33.

Bennett, J. A. 1995. Methodological notes on empathy: Further considerations. *Advances in Nursing Science* 18:36–50.

Beresford, A. 2005. Translator's Introduction. *Protagoras and Meno,* translated by A. Beresford. London: Penguin Classics, pp. xii–xxiv.

Bishop, S. 1992. Guidelines for a non-sexist (gender-sensitive) doctor-patient relationship. *Canadian Journal of Psychiatry* 37:62–5.

Bloch, S., and P. Chodoff, eds. 1981. *Psychiatric ethics.* Oxford: Oxford University Press.

Bloch, S., Chodoff, P., and S. Green, eds. 1999. *Psychiatric ethics, third edition.* Oxford: Oxford University Press.

Bloch, S., and R. Pargiter. 1999. Codes of ethics in psychiatry. In *Psychiatric ethics, third edition,* ed. S. Bloch, P. Chodoff, and S. Green, 81–103. Oxford: Oxford University Press.

Bloch, S., and S. Green. 2006. An ethical framework for psychiatry. *British Journal of Psychiatry* 188:7–12.

Blum, L. 1980. *Friendship, altruism, and morality.* London: Routledge.

Blum, L. 1986. Compassion. In *Explaining emotions,* ed. A. Rorty, 507–17. Berkeley: University of California Press.

Blum, L. 2007. Racial virtues. In *Working virtue,* eds. Walker and Ivanhoe, 225–250. Oxford: Oxford University Press.

Bolin, A. 1994. Transcending and transgendering: Male-to-female transsexuals, dichotomy and diversity. In *Third sex third gender: Beyond sexual dimorphism in culture and history,* ed. E. Herdt, 447–86. New York: Zone Books.

Borstein, K. 1994. *Gender outlaw: On men, women and the rest of us.* London: Routledge.

Bracken, P., and P. Thomas. 2005. *Postpsychiatry: Mental health in a postmodern world.* Oxford: Oxford University Press.

Brendel, D. 2006. *Healing psychiatry.* Cambridge, MA: MIT Press.

Brennan, S. 1999. Recent work in feminist ethics. *Ethics* 109:858–93.

Brothers, L. 1989. A biological perspective on empathy. *American Journal of Psychiatry* 146:1.

Broverman, I. K., Broverman, D. M., Clarkson, F. E., Rosenkrantz, P. S., and S. R. Vogel. 1970. Sex-role stereotypes and clinical judgments of mental health. *Journal of Counseling and Clinical Psychology* 34:1–7.

Brown, L. 1994. *Subversive dialogues: Theory in feminist therapy.* New York: Basic Books.

Burton, R. 1948. *The anatomy of melancholy,* ed. F. Dell, and P. Jordan Smith. New York: Tudor.

Burnyeat, M. F. 1980. Learning to be Good. In *Essays on Aristotle's ethics* ed., A. Rorty. 69–92. Berkeley, CA: University of California Press.

Busfield, J. 1986. *Managing madness: Changing ideas and practice.* London: Routledge.

Busfield, J. 1996. *Men, women and madness: Understanding gender and mental disorder.* New York: New York University Press.

Calhoun, C. 1995. Standing for something. *Journal of Philosophy* 92:235–60.

Campbell, A. V. 2003. The virtues and vices of the four principles. *Journal of Medical Ethics* 29:292–96.

Campbell, P. 1996. Challenging loss of power. In *Speaking our minds: An anthology*, ed. J. Read and J. Reynolds, 56–62. London: Macmillan.

Candilis, P., Martinez, R., and C. Dording. 2001. Principles and narrative in forensic psychiatry: Toward a robust view of professional role. *Journal of the American Academy of Psychiatry and Law* 29:167–73.

Caplan, P., and M. Gans. 1991. Is there empirical justification for the category of 'Self Defeating Personality Disorder'? *Feminism & Psychology* 1 (2):263–278.

Caplan, P. 1992. Driving us crazy: How oppression damages women's mental health and what we can do about it. *Women & Therapy* 12 (3):5–28.

Caplan, P. 1995a. *They say you're crazy.* New York: Addison-Wesley Publishing Company.

Caplan, P. 1995b. How *do* they decide who is normal? The bizarre, but true, tale of the DSM process. *Canadian Psychology* 32:162–70.

Card, C., ed. 1991. *Feminist ethics.* Lawrence: University of Kansas Press.

Chambers, T. 1999. *The fiction of bioethics.* New York: Routledge.

Charland, L., and P. Dick. 1995. Should compassion be included in codes of ethics for physicians? *Annals of the Royal College of Physicians and Surgeons of Canada* 28 (7 October): 415–18.

Charlton, J. 1998. *Nothing about us without us.* Berkeley: University of California Press.

Champ, S. 1999. A most precious thread. *The Australia and New Zealand Journal of Mental Health Nursing* 7:54–59.

Charon, R. 2001. The patient-physician relationship. Narrative medicine: A model for empathy, reflection, profession, and trust. *Journal of the American Medical Association* 286 (15):1897–902.

Chervenak, F., and L. McCullough. 1995. The threat of the new managed practice of medicine to patient's autonomy. *Journal of Clinical Ethics* 6:320–23.

Chervenak, F., and L. McCullough. 2001. The moral foundation of medical leadership: The professional virtues of the physician as fiduciary of the patient. *American Journal of Obstetrics and Gynecology* 184:875–80.

Chowdhury, A. N. 1998. Hundred years of Koro in the history of a culture-bound syndrome. *International Journal of Social Psychiatry* 44 (3):181–88.

Christianson, R. 1994. The ethics of treating the untreatable. *Psychiatric Services* 46: 1217.

Christie, R., and C. Hoffmaster. 1986. *Ethical issues in family medicine.* New York: Oxford University Press.

Christman, J. 2004. Relational autonomy, liberal individualism and the social constitution of selves. *Philosophical Studies* 117:143–64.

Christman, J., and J. Anderson, eds. 2006. *Autonomy and the challenges to liberalism: New essays.* Chicago: University of Chicago Press.

Churchill, L. 1989. Reviving a distinctive medical ethics. *Hastings Center Report* 19 (3): 28–34.

Clouser, K. D., and B. Gert. 1994. A critique of principlism, and morality vs. principlism. In *Principles of health care ethics,* ed. R. Gillon and A. Lloyd, 251–66. London: John Wiley & Sons.

Compte-Spoonville, A. 2001. *A short treatise on the great virtues: The uses of philosophy in everyday life,* trans. C. Temerson. London: Heinemann.

Connell, R. 1995. *Masculinities.* Oxford: Polity Press.

Cooperstock, R. 1981. A review of women's psychotropic drug use. In *Women and mental health,* ed. E. Howell and M. Bayes, 131–40. New York: Basic Books.

Corring, D. *Being normal: Quality of life domains for people living with mental illness,* Ph.D. dissertation, London, Ontario, Canada, University of Western Ontario, Department of Rehabilitation Sciences, 2005.

Corrigan, P. W., and D. Penn. 1998. Disease and discrimination. *Journal of Mental Health* 6 (4):355–66.

Cox, D., La Caze, M., and M. P. Levine. 2003. *Integrity and the fragile self.* Burlington: Ashgate Press.

Crandall, C. 2004. Social contagion of binge eating. In *The interface of social and clinical psychology: Key readings,* ed. R. M. Kowalsky and M. R. Leary, 99–115. New York: Psychology Press.

Crisp, R. 1992. Utilitarianism and the life of virtue. *Philosophical Quarterly* 167:139–60.

Crisp, R., ed. 1996. *How should one live?: Essays on the virtues.* Oxford: Oxford University Press.

Crisp, R., and Cowton, C. 1994. Hypocrisy and moral seriousness. *American Philosophical Quarterly* 31:343–49.

Crisp, R., and M. Slote. 1997. Introduction. In *Virtue Ethics,* ed. R. Crisp and M. Slote, 1–25. Oxford: Oxford University Press.

Crowden, A. 2003. Ethically sensitive mental health care. *The Australian and New Zealand Journal of Psychiatry* 17 (2):143–49.

Custance, J. 1952. *Wisdom, madness and folly.* New York: Farrar, Straus & Cudahy, Inc.

Curzer, H. 1993. Is care a virtue for healthcare professionals? *Journal of Medicine and Philosophy* 18 (1):51–69.

Dain, N. 1999. Reflections on antipsychiatry and stigma in the history of American psychiatry. *American Journal of Psychiatry* 45 (10):1010–15.

Davidson, L., and T. H. McGlashen. 1997. The varied outcomes of schizophrenia. *Canadian Journal of Psychiatry* 42 (1):34–43.

Davidson, L. 2003. *Living outside mental illness: Qualitative studies of recovery in schizophrenia.* New York: New York University Press.

Davis, M. H. 1994. *Empathy: A social psychological approach.* Madison: Brown and Benchmark Publishers.

Dawes, R. 1994. *House of cards: Psychology and psychotherapy built on myth.* New York: The Free Press.

Deegan, P. E. 1996. Recovery and the conspiracy of hope. http://www.patdeegan.com/aboutus_paper.html. Last accessed September 9, 2008.

Deigh, J. 1995. Empathy and universalizability. *Ethics* 105:4.

De Raeve, L. 1996. Caring intensively. In *Philosophical problems in healthcare*, ed. D. Greaves and H. Upton, 19–20. Aldershott: Avebury.

Dickenson, D., and K. W. M. Fulford. 2000. *In two minds: A casebook of psychiatric ethics.* Oxford: Oxford University Press.

Dillon, R. S., ed. 1995. *Dignity, character, and self-respect.* London: Routledge.

Doris, J. 2002. *Lack of character: Personality and moral behavior.* Cambridge: Cambridge University Press.

Drane, J. 1995. *Becoming a good doctor: The place of virtue and character in medical ethics, second edition.* Kansas City: Sheed and Ward.

Driver, J. 1996. The virtues and human nature. In *How should one live?: Essays on the virtues*, ed. R. Crisp, 111–29. Oxford: Oxford University Press.

Dunn, C. 1998. *Ethical issue in mental illness.* Aldershot: Avebury.

Dyer, A. 1988. *Ethics and psychiatry: Toward professional definition.* Washington, DC: American Psychiatric Press.

Dyer, A. 1999. Psychiatry as a profession. In *Psychiatric ethics, third edition*, ed. S. Bloch, P. Chodoff and S. A.Green, 67–79. Oxford: Oxford University Press.

Edelwich, J., and Brodsky, A. 1991. *Sexual dilemmas for the helping professional.* New York: Brunner.

Edwards, R., ed. 1982. *Ethics of psychiatry: Insanity, rational autonomy, and mental health care.* New York: Prometheus Books.

Edwards, R., ed. 1997. *Ethics of psychiatry: Insanity, rational autonomy, and mental health care, second edition.* New York: Prometheus Books.

Elkin, I., Shea, M. T., Watkins, J. T., et al. 1989. NIMH treatment of depression collaborative research program: General effectiveness of treatments. *Archives of General Psychiatry* 46:971–82.

Elkin, I., Parloff, M. B., Hadley, S. W., and J. H. Autry. 1985. NIMH Treatment of depression collaborative research program: Background and research plan. *Archives of General Psychiatry* 42:305–16.

Elkin, I., Pilkonis, M. B., Docherty, J. P., and S. M. Sotsky. 1985. Conceptual and methodological issues in comparative studies of the psychotherapy and psychopharmacotherapy. 1: Active Ingredients and Mechanism of Change *American Journal of Psychiatry* 145:909–17.

Elkin, I., Pilkonis, M. B., Docherty, J. P., and S. M. Sotsky. 1985. 2: Nature and timing of treatment effects. *American Journal of Psychiatry* 145:1070–76.

Elkin, I., Pilkonis, M. B., Docherty, J. P., and S. M. Sotsky. 1989. NIMH treatment of depression collaborative research program: General effectiveness of treatments. *Archives of General Psychiatry* 46:971–82.

Ekins, R., and D. King. 1997. Blending genders: Contributions to the emerging field of transgender studies. *International Journal of Transgenderism* 1 (1). http://www.symposion.com/ijk/ihtco101.htm.

Elliott, C. 1999. *Bioethics, culture and identity: A philosophical disease.* New York: Routledge.

Elliott, C., and P. Kramer. 2003. *Better than well: American medicine meets the American dream.* New York: W. W. Norton & Co.

Elshtain, J. B. 1987. Against androgyny. In *Feminism and equality,* ed. A. Phillips, 139–59. Oxford: Oxford University Press.

Emanuel, L., and E. Emanuel. 1992. Four models of the physician-patient relationship. *Journal of the American Medical Association* 267 (16):2221–26.

Erwin, E. 1978. *Behavior therapy: Scientific, philosophical and moral foundations.* New York: Cambridge University Press.

Erwin, E. 2004. Cognitive-behavioral therapy. In *The philosophy of psychiatry: A companion,* ed. J. Radden, 381–92. New York: Oxford University Press.

Everett, B. 2000. *A fragile revolution: Consumers and psychiatric survivors confront the power of the mental health system.* Waterloo: Wilfrid Laurier University Press.

Ewing, C. P., and J. T. McCann. 2006. *Minds on trial: Great cases in law and psychology.* Oxford: Oxford University Press.

Exdell, J. 1987. Ethics, ideology, and feminine virtue. In *Science, morality and feminist theory,* ed. M. Hanen and K. Nielsen, 169–99. Calgary: University of Calgary Press.

Fabrega, H., Jr. 1990. Psychiatric stigma in the classical and medieval period: A review of the literature. *Comprehensive Psychiatry* 31 (4):289–306.

Fabrega, H., Jr. 1991. The culture and history of psychiatric stigma in early modern and modern western societies: A review of recent literature. *Comprehensive Psychiatry* 32 (2):97–119.

Fausto-Sterling, A. 2000. *Sexing the body: Gender politics and the construction of sexuality.* New York: Basic Books.

Feder, E. 1997. Disciplining the family: The case of gender identity disorder *Philosophical Studies* 85:195–211.

Feinberg, L. 1996. *Transgender warriors.* Boston: Beacon Press.

Feinberg, L. 1998. *Trans liberation: Beyond pink or blue.* Boston: Beacon.

Ferguson, A. 1977. Androgyny as an ideal of human development. In *Feminism and philosophy* ed. M. Vetterling-Braggin, M. Elliston, and J. English, 45–69. Totowa: Rowman.

Flanagan, O., and A. Rorty. 1990. *Identity, character and morality.* Cambridge: MIT Press.

Flexner, A. 1915. Is social work a profession? *Proceedings of the National Conference of Charities and Corrections,* Baltimore, MD: Chicago: National Conference of Charities and Corrections, 42nd Meeting, Baltimore, MD, May 12–19, 1915.

Foot, P. 1978. *Virtues and vices.* Berkeley: University of California Press.

Foucault, M. 1971. *Madness and civilization: A history of insanity in the age of reason,* trans. R. Howard. New York: Vintage.

Frader, J., Alderson, P., Asch, A., et al. 2004. Health care professionals and intersex conditions. *Archives of Pediatric Adolescent Medicine* 158:426–29.

Frank, J., and B. Frank. 1991. *Persuasion and healing, third edition.* Baltimore: Johns Hopkins University Press.

Frank, E., ed. 2000. *Gender and its effects on psychopathology.* Washington, DC: American Psychiatric Press.

Fraser, A. 2000. *Ethics for psychiatrists derived from virtue theory.* Lecture delivered at Fourth International Conference on Philosophy and Mental Health, Florence (Italy), August 2000.

Fraser, N. 2003. Social justice in the age of identity politics: Redistribution, recognition, and participation. In *Redistribution or recognition?: A political-philosophical exchange,* ed. N. Fraser and A. Honneth, 7–109. London: Verso.

Freedman, A. M., and A. L. Halpern. 1996. The erosion of ethics and morality in medicine: Physician participation in legal executions in the United States. *New York Law School Law Review* 41 (1):169–88.

Freedman, A. M., and J. Radden. 2006. Judicial uses for forced psychotropic medication. *International Journal of Mental Health* 35 (1):3–11.

Freeman, L., and J. Roy. 1976. *Betrayal.* New York: Stein and Day.

Freud, S. 1959. *Collected papers of Sigmund Freud,* trans. J. Rivière. London: Hogarth Press.

Fried, C. 1976. The lawyer as friend: The moral foundations of the lawyer-client relation. *Yale Law Journal* 85 (2):1060.

Friedman, M. 2003. *Autonomy, gender, politics.* New York: Oxford University Press.

Fulford, K. W. M. 1989. *Moral theory and medical practice.* Cambridge: Cambridge University Press.

Fulford K. W. M, Smirnov, A. Y., and E. Snow. 1993. Concepts of disease and the abuse of psychiatry in the USSR. *British Journal of Psychiatry* 162:801–10.

Fulford, K. W. M., and T. Hope. 1994. Psychiatric ethics: A bioethical ugly duckling? In *Principles of healthcare ethics,* ed. R. Gillon. London: John Wiley & Sons.

Fulford, K. W. M., Morris, K., Stanghellini, G., and J. Sadler, eds. 2003. *Nature and narrative: An introduction to the new philosophy of psychiatry.* Oxford, UK: Oxford University Press.

Fulford, K. W. M. 2004. Facts/values: Ten principles of values-based medicine. In *The philosophy of psychiatry: A companion,* ed. J. Radden, 205–34. Oxford and New York: Oxford University Press.

Gabbard, G. 1989. *Sexual exploitation in professional relationships.* Washington, DC: American Psychiatric Press.

Gabbard, G. 1999. Boundary violations. In *Psychiatric ethics*, ed. S. Bloch, P. Chodoff, and S. Green, 141–60. Oxford: Oxford University Press.

Gaines, A. D. 1992. From DSM-I to III-R; Voices of self, mastery, and the other: A cultural constructivist reading of U. S. psychiatric classification. *Social Science and Medicine* 35 (1): 3–24.

Gallese, V. 2003. The manifold nature of interpersonal relations: The quest for a common mechanism. *Philosophical Transactions of the Royal Society of London Series B* 358:517–28.

Gantrell, N.,ed. 1994. *Bringing ethics alive: Feminist ethics in psychotherapeutic practice.* New York: Haworth Press.

Garber, M. 1996. *Vice versa: Bisexuality and the eroticism of everyday life.* London: Hamish Hamilton.

Gardner, H. 1993. *Multiple intelligences: The theory in practice.* New York: Basic Books.

Gehring, V. V. 2003. Phonies, fakes and frauds—and the social harm they cause. *Philosophy & Public Policy Quarterly* 23 (1–2):14–20.

Gert, B., Clouser, K. D., and C. M. Culver. 1997. *Bioethics: A return to fundamentals.* New York: Oxford University Press.

Ghaemi, S. N. 2003. *The concepts of psychiatry: Toward understanding the mind and its pathologies.* Baltimore: Johns Hopkins Press.

Gilligan, C. 1982. *In a different voice.* Cambridge: Harvard University Press.

Gilman, S. 1982. *Seeing the insane.* New York: John Wiley & Sons.

Glover, J. 2003. Towards humanism in psychiatry. Tanner Lectures, Princeton University, February 12–14, 2003. http://www.tannerlectures.utah.edu/lectures/documents/volume24/glover_2003.pdf. Last accessed September 9, 2008.

Goleman, D. 1995. *Emotional intelligence: It can matter more than IQ.* New York: Bantom Books.

Goodin, R. E. 1988. Reasons for welfare: Economic, sociological, and political—But ultimately moral. In *Responsibility, rights and welfare*, ed. J. D. Moon, 37. Boulder Colorado: Westview Press.

Gordon, R. 1995. Sympathy, simulation, and the impartial spectator. *Ethics* 105 (4): 743–63.

Gottlieb, P. 1994. Aristotle's 'nameless' virtues. *Apeiron* 27(1):1–15.

Goulet, J.-G. 2001. The 'Berdache'/two spirit: A comparison of anthropological and native constructions of gendered identities among the Northern Athapaskans. *Journal of the Royal Anthropology Institute* 2:683–701.

Green, S. 1999. The ethics of managed mental health care. In *Psychiatric ethics, third edition*, ed. S. Bloch, P. Chodoff, and S. A. Green, 401–21. Oxford: Oxford University Press.

Green, S., and S. Bloch. 2001. Working in a flawed mental health care system: An ethical challenge. *American Journal of Psychiatry* 158:1378–83.

Gutheil, T., and G. Gabbard. 1998. Misuses and misunderstandings of boundary theory in clinical and regulatory settings. *American Journal of Psychiatry* 155 (3):409–14.

Guze, S. B. 1989. Biological psychiatry: Is there any other kind? *Psychological Medicine* 19 (2):315–23.

Halpern, J. 2001. *From detached concern to empathy: Humanizing medical practice.* New York: Oxford University Press.

Hardimon, M. 1994. Role obligations. *The Journal of Philosophy* XCI (7):333–63.

Harris, G. W. 1979. *Dignity and vulnerability: Strengths and quality of character.* Berkeley: University of California Press.

Havens, L. 1987. *Approaches to the mind: Movements of the psychiatric schools from sects toward science.* Cambridge: Harvard University Press.

Heilbrun, C. 1980. Androgyny and the future of sex differences. In *The future of difference,* ed. H. Eisenstein, and A. Jardine,258–66. Boston: Harvard University Press.

Henderson, A. 2001. Emotional labor and nursing: An under-appreciated aspect of caring work. *Nursing Inquiry* 8 (2):130–38.

Herdt, G. 1994. *Third sex third gender: Beyond sexual dimorphism in culture and history.* New York: Zone Books.

Herman, B. 1993. *The practice of moral judgement.* Cambridge: Harvard University Press.

Heyd, D. 2006. Superogation. In *The Stanford encyclopedia of philosophy,* ed. E N. Zalta, *http://plato.stanford.edu/entries/supererogation/* Last accessed September 9, 2008.

Hirshbein, L. D. 2006. Science, gender, and the emergence of depression in American psychiatry, 1952–1980. *Journal of the History of Medicine and Allied Sciences* 67 (2): 187–216.

Holmes, J., and R. Lindley. 1989. *The values of psychotherapy.* Oxford: Oxford University Press.

Hoffman, M. L. 1984. Empathy, its limitations and its role in a comprehensive moral theory. In *Moral behavior and development: Advances in theory, research, and applications,* ed. W. Kurtines and J. Gerwitz, 283–302. New York: John Wiley and Sons.

Hoffman, M. L. 2000. *Empathy and moral development: Implications for caring and justice.* Cambridge: Cambridge University Press.

Horwitz, A. 2002. *Creating mental illness.* Chicago: Chicago University Press.

Hume, D. 1965. *A treatise of human nature.* Oxford: Clarendon Press.

Hurley, S., and N. Chater, eds. 2005. *From neuroscience to social science.* Cambridge: MIT Press.

Hursthouse, R. 1999. *On virtue ethics*. Oxford: Oxford University Press.

Ickes, W., ed. 1997. *Empathy accuracy*. New York: Guilford Press.

Illingworth, P. 1988. The friendship model of physician/patient relationship and patient autonomy. *Bioethics* 2 (1):22–36.

IBGR. 1995. International Bill of Gender Rights. http://www.pfc.org.uk/node/275. Laset Accessed September 23, 2006.

Irigaray, L. 1985. *This sex which is not one*, trans. C. Porter. Ithaca: Cornell University Press.

Irving, P., and D. Dickson. 2004. Empathy: Towards a conceptual framework for health professionals. *International Journal of Health Care Quality Assurance Including Leadership in Health Services* 17 (4-5): 212–20.

Irwin, T. 1985. *Nichomachean ethics*, trans. T. Irwin. New York: Hackett.

Irwin, T. 1996. *Aristotle: Introductory readings*. Indianapolis: Hackett Publishing.

Isay, R. A. 1997. Remove gender identity disorder in DSM. *Psychiatric News* November 4:9.

Ivanhoe, P., and B. Van Norden, ed. 2001. *Readings in classical Chinese philosophy*. Indiapolis: Hackett.

Jackson S. 1999. *Care of the psyche: A history of psychological healing*. New Haven: Yale University Press.

Jacobson, N., and J. Greenley. 2001. What is recovery? A conceptual model and explication. *Psychiatric Services* 52 (4):482–85.

Jamison, K. R. 1995. *An unquiet mind*. New York: Knopf.

Jordan, J., Surrey, J., Kaplan, A., and J. B. Miller. 1991. *Women's growth in connection: Writings from the Stone Center*. New York: The Guilford Press.

Karasu, T. 1999. Ethical aspects of psychotherapy. In *Psychiatric Ethics* edited by Bloch, S., Chodoff, P., and Green, S.89–116. Oxford: Oxford University Press.

Kant, I. 1978. *Anthropology from a pragmatic point of view*, trans. V. Dowdell. Carbondale: Southern Illinois University Press.

Kaplan, B., ed. 1964. *The inner world of mental illness*. New York: Harper & Row.

Kaplan, H., and B. Sadock. 1995. *Comprehensive textbook of psychiatry*. Volumes 1 & 2. 6th edition. Baltimore: Williams & Wilkins.

Karr, M. D. 1994. Acting in medical practice. *Lancet* 43 (4): 1436.

Katz, J. 1990. The invention of heterosexuality. *Socialist Review* 20:7–34.

Katz, J. 1995. *The invention of heterosexuality*. New York: Dutton.

Kempe, M. 1985. *The book of Margery Kempe*, trans. B. A. Windeatt. London: Penguin Books.

Kessler, R. C., McGonigle, K. A., Zhao, S., et al. 1994. Lifetime and 12 month prevalence of DSM-III-R psychiatric disorders in the United States. Results from the National Comorbidity Survey. *Archives of General Psychiatry* 51 (1):8–19.

Kessler, S. 1998. *Lessons from the intersexed*. New Brunswick: Rutgers University Press.

Kittay, E. 1982. On hyprocisy. *Metaphilosophy* 13:277–89.

Kramer, P. 1993. *Listening to Prozac.* New York: Viking.

Korsgaard, C. 1996. *The sources of normativity.* Cambridge: Cambridge University Press.

Kroll, J. 2001. Boundary violations: A culture-bound syndrome. *Journal of the American Academy of Psychiatry and Law* 29 (3): 274–83.

Kronman, A. 1987. Living in the law. *University of Chicago Law Review* 54: 835–76.

Kopelman, L. 1999a. Help from Hume reconciling professionalism and managed care. *Journal of Medicine and Philosophy* 24 (4):396–410.

Kopelman L. 1999b. Values and virtues: How should they be taught? *Academic Medicine* 74 (12):1307–10.

Kupperman, J. J. 1991. *Character.* New York and Oxford: Oxford University Press.

Lazarus, J. A., and S. S. Shafstein, eds. 1998. *New roles for psychiatrists in organized systems of care.* Washington, DC: American Psychiatric Association Press.

Larson, E. B. 2003. Medicine as a profession—back to basics: Preserving the physician-patient relationship in a challenging medical marketplace. *American Journal of Medicine* 114: 168–72.

Larson, E. B., and Yao, X. Y. 2005. Clinical empathy as emotional labor in the patient-physician relationship. *Journal of the American Medical Association* 293 (9):1100–06.

Legato, M., ed. 2004. *Principles of gender-specific medicine.* New York: Academic Press.

Levenson, R., and A. Ruef. 1992. Empathy: A physiological substrate. *Journal of Personality and Social Psychology* 63 (2):234–46.

Lloyd, G. 1993. *The man of reason: "male" and "female" in western philosophy.* Minneapolis: University of Minnesota Press.

Lomas, P. 1999. *Doing good?: Psychotherapy out of its depth.* Oxford: Oxford University Press.

Luban, D., ed. 1984. *The good lawyer: Lawyer's roles and lawyer's ethics.* Totowa: Rowman and Allanheld.

Luhrmann, T. 2000. *Of two minds: The growing disorder in American psychiatry.* New York: Knopf.

Lunbeck, E. 1994. *The psychiatric persuasion: Knowledge, gender, and power in modern America.* Princeton: Princeton University Press.

Lustig, A. 1992. The method of 'principalism': A critique of the critique. *Journal of Medicine and Philosophy* 17:487–510.

Maccoby, E. E. 1998. *The two sexes: Growing up apart, coming together.* Cambridge, MA: Harvard University Press.

McKinnon, C. 1999. *Character, virtue theories and the vices.* Boulder: Broadview Press.

MacIntyre, A. 1984. *After virtue.* Notre Dame: University of Notre Dame Press.

MacIntyre, A. 1999. Social structures and their threats to moral agency. *Philosophy* 74 (289):311–29.

Mahowald, M. 1996. On treatment of myopia: Feminist standpoint theory and bioethics. In *Feminism and bioethics: Beyond reproduction*, ed. S. Wolf, 95–115. New York: Oxford University Press.

Mann, D. 1997. The virtues in psychiatric practice. *Theoretical Medicine* 18:21–30.

Martin, J. 1985. *Reclaiming a conversation: The ideal of the educated woman.* New Haven: Yale University Press.

Martin, N. 2001. Feminist bioethics and psychiatry. *Journal of Medicine and Philosophy* 26 (4):431–41.

Martinez, R. 2000. A model for boundary dilemmas: Ethical decision-making in the patient-professional relationship. *Ethical Human Sciences and Services* 2:43–61.

Matthews, D. A., A. L. Suchman, and W. T. Branch. 1993. Making "connecxions": Enhancing the therapeutic potential of patient-client relationships. *Annals of Internal Medicine* 118: 973–77.

May, W. 1983. *The physician's covenant: Images of the healer in medical ethics.* Philadelphia: The Westminster Press.

May, W. 1994. The virtues in a professional setting. In *Medicine and moral reasoning*, ed. K. W. M. Fulford, G. Gillett, and J. Martin Soskice, 75–90. Cambridge: Cambridge University Press.

Mayer, J., Salovey, P., and Carruso, D. R. 2000. Emotional intelligence as *Zeitgeist*, as personality, and as mental ability, in *The handbook of emotional intelligence*, ed. R. Bar-Ou, and J. Parker. San Francisco: Jossey-Bass, 92–117.

McFall, L. 1992. Integrity. In *Ethics and personality*, ed. J. Deigh, 79–94. Chicago: University of Chicago Press.

McDowell, J. 1979. Virtue and reason. *The Monist* 62 (3):49–72.

McHugh, P., and P. Slavney. 1987. *The perspectives of psychiatry, first edition.* Baltimore: Johns Hopkins Press.

McKeon, R. 1941. *Complete works of Aristotle.* New York: Random House.

McKinnon, C. 1991. Hypocrisy, with a note on integrity. *American Philosophical Quarterly* 28:321–30.

McKinnon, C. 1999. *Character, virtue theories and the vices.* Boulder: Broadview Press.

Mayer, R., and C. McLaughlan. 1998. *Between mind, brain, and managed care: The now and future world of academic psychiatry.* Washington, DC: American Psychiatric Press.

Metzger, W. P. 1975. What is a Profession? *Seminar reports, program of general and continuing education in the humanities* 3:1 New York: Columbia University, September 18, 1975: 1–12.

Megone, C. 2000. Mental illness, Human function, and values. *Philosophy, Psychiatry & Psychology* 7 (1):45–65.

Meyers, D., ed. 1997. *Feminists rethink the self.* Boulder: Westview Press.

Meyers, D. 2004. Narrative and moral life. In *Setting the moral compass: Essays by women philosophers,* ed. C. Calhoun, 288–305.

Miller, A. 2003. *An introduction to contemporary metaethics.* Cambridge: Polity.

Miller, J. B. 1976. *Toward a new psychology of women.* Boston: Beacon Press.

Miller, J. B., and Stiver, I. 1998. *The healing connection: How women form connections in both therapy and in life.* Boston: Beacon Press.

Minogue, B. 2000. The two fundamental duties of the physician. *Academic Medicine* 75 (5):431–42.

Moerman, D. 2002. *Meaning, medicine and the 'placebo effect'.* Cambridge: Cambridge University Press.

Morgan, K. 2002. Gender police. In *Foucault and the Government of Disability,* ed. S. Tremain, 298–328. Ann Arbor Michigan: University of Michigan Press.

Moore, M., and M. Sparrow. 1990. *Ethics in government: The moral challenge of public leadership.* Englewood CliffsJ: Prentice-Hall.

Morreim, E. H. 1990. The new economics of medicine: Special changes to psychiatry. *Journal of Medicine and Philosophy* 15:98.

Morris, S. 2000. Heaven is a mad place on earth. In *Mad pride: A celebration of mad culture,* ed. T. Curtis, R. Dellar, E. Leslie, and B. Watson, 207–08. London: Spare Change Books.

Murdoch, I. 1967. *The sovereignty of the good.* Cambridge: Cambridge University Press.

Musto, D. F. 1999. A historical perspective. In *Psychiatric ethics,* ed. S. Bloch, P. Chodoff, S. Green, 7–24. Oxford: Oxford University Press.

Nanda, S. 1989. *Neither man nor woman: The Hijras of India.* Belmont: Wadsworth.

National Bioethics Advisory Commission. 1998. Research Involving Persons with Mental Disorders That May Affect Decisionmaking Capacity, December 1998. Washington, DC: National Bioethics Advisory Commission. http://bioethics.gov/pubs.html. Last accessed June 6, 2005.

Nelson, J. L. 2003. *Rationing sanity: Ethical issues in managed mental health care.* Washington, DC: Georgetown University Press.

Nelson, H. L. 2001. *Damaged identities: Narrative repair.* Ithaca: Cornell University Press.

Nissim-Sabat, M. 2004. Race and culture. In *The philosophy of psychiatry: A companion,* ed. J. Radden, 244–57. New York: Oxford University Press.

Neugeboren, J. 1999. *Transforming madness: New lives for people living with mental illness.* Berkeley: University of California Press.

Nussbaum, M. 1996. *Upheavals of thought: A theory of the emotions.* Gifford Lectures 1993. Cambridge and New York: Cambridge University Press.

Nussbaum, M. 1999. Virtue ethics: A misleading category. *Ethics* 3 (3):1382–4554.

Oakley, J. 1996. Varieties of virtue. *Ethics* IX (2):128–52.

Oakley J., and D. Cocking. 2001. *Virtue ethics and professional roles*. Cambridge: Cambridge University Press.

Okin, S. M. 1989. *Justice, gender and the family*. New York: Basic Books.

Okin, S. M. 1996. Feminism, moral development and the virtues. In *How Should One Live?: Essays on the Virtues,* ed. R. Crisp, 211–29. Oxford: Oxford University Press.

Oyewumi, O. 1997. *The invention of women: Making an African sense of western gender discourses*. Minneapolis: University of Minnesota Press.

Ozar, D. T. 1995. Profession and professional ethics. In *Encyclopedia of Bioethics, revised edition*, ed. W. T. Reich, 2103–12. New York: Simon and Schuster.

Parsons, T. 1951. *The social system*. Chicago, Illinois: The Free Press.

Pellegrino, E. 1979. Toward a reconstruction of medical morality: The primacy of the act of profession and the fact of illness. *Journal of Medicine and Philosophy* 4 (1):32–56.

Pellegrino, E., and Thomasma, D. 1993. *The virtues of medical practice*. New York: Oxford University Press.

Percival, T. 1803. *Code of medical ethics; or a code of institutes and precepts, adapted to the professional conduct of physicians and surgeons*. Manchester: S. Russell.

Pence, G. 1991. Virtue theory. In *A companion to ethics*, ed. P. Singer, 249–58. Oxford: Blackwell.

Peplau. L. 2003. Human sexuality: How do men and women differ? *Current Directions in Psychological Science* 12:37–44.

Peterson, C., and M. Seligman. 2004. *Character strengths and virtues: A handbook and classification*. Oxford: Oxford University Press.

Phillips, J. 1980–81. Transference and countertransference: The therapeutic relationship in psychoanalytic and existential psychotherapy. *Review of Existential Psychology & Psychiatry* 17 (2–3):135–52.

Pickering, N. 2006. *The metaphor of mental illness*. Oxford: Oxford University Press.

Pincoffs, E. 1986. *Quandaries and virtues: Against reductivism in ethics*. Lawrence: University of Kansas Press.

Plaut, S. M. 1997. Boundary violations in professional-client relationships: Overview and guidelines of prevention. *Sexual and Marital Therapy* 12 (1):77–94.

Poland, J., Von Eckhardt, B., and W. Spaulding. 1994. Problems with the DSM approach to classifying psychopathology. In *Philosophical psychopathology*, ed. G. Graham and G. L. Stephens, 235–60. Cambridge: The MIT Press.

Postema, G. 1980. Moral responsibility in professional ethics. *New York University Law Review* 55 (1): 63–89.

Potter, N. N. 2002. *How can I be trusted? A virtue theory of trustworthiness*. New York: Rowman & Littlefield Publishers Inc.

Potter, N. 2004. Gender. In *Philosophy of psychiatry: A companion*, ed. J. Radden, 237–43. New York and Oxford: Oxford University Press.

Povar, G J., Blumen, H., Daniel, J., et al. 2004. Medicine as a profession managed care ethics working group. *Annals of Internal Medicine* 141 (2):131–36.

Prinz, J. 2005. Imitation and moral development. In *From neuroscience to social science, volume I and II*, ed. S. Hurley, and N. Chater, 267–282. Cambridge: MIT Press.

Prior, P. 1999. *Gender and mental health*. New York: New York University Press.

Quadrio, C. 2001. *Women working and training in Australian psychiatry*. Sydney: Book House.

Radden, J. 1996. Relational individualism and feminist therapy. *Hypatia* 11:72–96.

Radden, J., ed. 2000. *The nature of melancholy: From Aristotle to Kristeva*. New York: Oxford University Press.

Radden, J. 2001. Boundary violation ethics: Some conceptual clarifications. *Journal of the American Academy of Psychiatry and Law* 29 (3):319–26.

Radden, J. 2002a. Notes towards a professional ethics for psychiatry. *Australian & New Zealand Journal of Psychiatry* 36 (2):52–9.

Radden, J. 2002b. Background briefing on psychiatric ethics. *Bioethics* 16 (5):397–411.

Radden, J. 2003. Forced medication, patients' rights and values conflicts. *Psychiatry, Psychology, and Law* 10 (1):1–11.

Radden, J., ed. 2004. *Philosophy of psychiatry: A companion*. New York and Oxford: Oxford University Press.

Radden, J. 2007. My symptoms, myself: Reading mental illness memoirs for identity assumptions. In *Depression and narrative*, ed. H. Clarke, 15–28. New York: SUNY Press.

Radden, J. 2008. Thinking about the repair manual: Technique and technology in psychiatry. In *Philosophical perspectives on psychiatry and technology*, ed. J. Phillips, 263–78. Oxford, UK: Oxford University Press.

Radden J., and J. Sadler. 2008. Character virtues in psychiatric practice. *Harvard Review of Psychiatry* 16 (6): 373–80.

Railton, P. 1988. How thinking about character and utilitarianism might lead to rethinking the character of utilitarianism. In *Midwest Studies in Philosophy XIII*, ed. P. French, T. Uehling, and H. Wettstein, 398–415. Indianna: The University of Notre Dame.

Rajczi, A. 2003. Why are there no expert teachers of virtue? *Educational Theory* 53 (4):389–400.

Ramet, S. P. 1 996. *Gender reversals and gender cultures: Anthropological and historical perspectives*. London: Routledge.

Read, J., and J. Reynolds, eds. 1996. *Speaking our minds: An anthology*. London: Macmillan Press.

Rieff, P. 1959. *Freud: the mind of the moralist*. London: Methuen and Co., Ltd.

Reiser, S., Bursztajn, H., Appelbaum, P., and T. Gutheil. 1987. *Divided staffs, divided selves: A case approach to mental health ethics*. Cambridge: Cambridge University Press.

Reich, W. 1999. Psychiatric diagnosis as an ethical problem. In *Psychiatric ethics, third edition*, ed. S. Bloch, P. Chodoff and S. A. Green. Oxford: Oxford University Press.

Rest, J. 1986. *Moral development: Advances in theory and research.* New York: Praeger.

Rhodes, R. 2005. Rethinking research ethics. *American Journal of Bioethics* 5 (1):7–28.

Richardson, F., Flowers, B., and C. Guignon. 1999. *Re-envisioning psychology: Moral dimensions in theory and practice.* San Francisco: Jossey-Bass.

Ridgeway, P. 2001. Re-storying psychiatric disability: Learning from first-person narrative accounts of recovery. *Psychiatric Rehabilitation Journal* 24 (4):335–43.

Robb, C. 2007. *This changes everything: The relational revolution in psychology.* New York: Farrar, Straus, and Giroux.

Roberts, L. W., and B. Roberts. 1999. Psychiatric research ethics: An overview of evolving guidelines and current ethical dilemmas in the study of mental illness. *Biological Psychiatry* 46:1025–38.

Robins, L., and D. Regier, eds. 1991. *Psychiatric disorders in America: the epidemiologic catchment area study.* New York: Free Press.

Rogers, C. 1957. The necessary and sufficient conditions of therapeutic personality change. *Journal of Consulting Psychology* 21:95–103.

Rosenthal, E. 2003. How doctors learn to think they're doctors. *New York Times,* November 28.

Roscoe, W. 1991. *The Zuni Man-Woman.* Albuquerque: U of New Mexico press.

Rossler, B. 2002. Problems with autonomy. *Hypatia* 17 (4):143–162.

Ruddick, S. 1995. *Maternal thinking: Toward a politics of peace.* Boston: Beacon Press.

Russell, D. 1994. Psychiatric diagnosis and the interests of women. In *Philosophical perspectives on psychiatric diagnostic classification*, ed. J. Z. Sadler, O. P. Wiggins, and M. A. Schwartz, 246–59. Baltimore: The Johns Hopkins University Press.

Sabin, J. E. 1994. Caring about patients and caring about money: the American Psychiatric Association code of ethics meets managed care. *Behavioral Sciences & the Law* 12 (4):317–30.

Sabin, J. E. 1995. General hospital psychiatry and the ethics of managed care. *General Hospital Psychiatry* 17 (4):293–98.

Sadler, J. Z. 1986. The emergency room psychiatrist as multiple agent: A family systems analysis. *Family Systems Medicine* 4 (4):367–375.

Sadler, J. Z. 2002. *Descriptions and prescriptions: Values, mental disorders, and the DSMs.* Baltimore: The Johns Hopkins University Press.

Sadler, J. Z. 2003. Mental illness, III: Issues in diagnosis. In *Encyclopedia of bioethics, third edition*, ed. S. E. Post, 1810–1815. New York: MacMillan Reference.

Sadler, J. Z. 2004. Diagnosis and anti-diagnosis. *In Philosophy of psychiatry: A companion*, ed. J. Radden, 163–79. New York and Oxford: Oxford University Press.

Sadler, J. Z. 2005. *Values and psychiatric diagnosis.* Oxford: Oxford University Press.

Sadler, J. Z. 2007. The psychiatric significance of the personal self. *Psychiatry* 70 (2):113–29.

Sadler, J. Z, Wiggins, O. P., and M. A. Schwartz. 1994. Introduction. In *Philosophical perspectives on psychiatric diagnostic classification*, ed. J. Z. Sadler, O. P. Wiggins, and M. A. Schwartz. Baltimore: Johns Hopkins University Press.

Salovey, P., and J. D. Mayer. 1990. Emotional intelligence. *Imagination, cognition, and personality* 9:185–211.

Schechtman, M. 1996. *The constitution of selves*. New Work: Columbia University Press.

Scheler, M. 1970. *The nature of sympathy*. Hamden: Shoe String.

Scheman, N. 1997. Queering the center by centering the queer: Reflections on transsexuals and secular Jews. In *Feminists rethink the self*, ed. D. Meyers, 124–62. Boulder: Westview Press.

Schlesinger, M., Wynia, M., and D. Cummins. 2000. Some distinctive features of the impact of managed care on psychiatry. *Harvard Review of Psychiatry* 8:216–30.

Schreber, D. 1988. Memoirs of my nervous illness, trans. I. MacAlpine and R. M. Hunter. Cambridge: Harvard University Press.

Sedgwick, P. 1982. *Psycho politics*. New York: Harper and Row.

Shapiro, J. 1990. Patterns of psychosocial performance in the doctor-patient encounter: A study of family practice residents. *Social Science & Medicine* 31 (9):35–141.

Shapiro, J., E. Morrison, and J. R. Baker. 2004. Teaching empathy to first-year medical students: Evaluation of an elective literature and medicine course. *Education for Health* 17 (1), 74–84.

Shea, M. T., Elkin, I., and Imber, S. D., et al. 1992. Course of depressive symptoms over follow up: Findings from the NIMH treatment of depression collaborative research program. *Archives of General Psychiatry* 49:782–87.

Sherwin, S. 1992. *Patient no more*. Philadelphia: Temple University Press

Shorter, E. 1997. *A history of psychiatry: From the era of the asylum to the age of prozac*. New York: John Wiley & Sons.

Showalter, E. 1986. *The female malady*. Princeton: Princeton University Press.

Simon. R. T. 1992. Treatment boundary violations: Clinical, ethical, and legal considerations. *Bulletin of the American Academy of Psychiatry* 20:269–88.

Skultans, V. 1979. *English madness: Ideas on insanity 1550–1890*. London: Routledge & Kegan Paul.

Slater, L. 1998. *Prozac diary*. New York: Penguin Books.

Sloane R. B., Staples, F. R., Cristol, A. H., Yorkston, N. J., and K. Whipple. 1975. *Psychotherapy versus behavior therapy*. Cambridge: Harvard University Press.

Slote, M. 2003. Sentimentalist virtue and moral judgment: Outline of a project. *Metaphilosophy* 34 (1–2): 131–43.

Slote, M. 2004. *Ethical theory and moral practice*. New York: Springer.

Smith, B. G., and E. Hutchinson, eds. 2004. *Gendering disability*. New Brunswick, NJ: Rutgers University Press.

Soble, J. 2004. Paraphilias and distress in DSM-IV. In *A companion to the philosophy of psychiatry*, ed. J. Radden, 54–63. Oxford: Oxford University Press.

Sotsky, S. M., Glass, D. R., Shea, M. T., et al. 1991. Patient predictors of response to psychotherapy and pharmacotherapy: Findings of the NIMH treatment of depression collaborative research program. *American Journal of Psychiatry* 148:997–1008.

Spitz, D. 1996. Collaboration between psychiatrist and patient: How avoidable is paternalism? *Annual Review of Law and Ethics* 4:233–248.

Stack Sullivan, H. 1954. *The psychiatric interview*. New York: W. W. Norton.

Stark, A. 1995. The appearance of official impropriety and the concept of political crime. *Ethics* 105:326–351.

Sternberg, R., ed. 2000. *Handbook of intelligence*. Cambridge: Cambridge University Press.

Stohr, K., and C. H. Wellman. 2002. Recent Work in virtue ethics. *American Philosophical Quarterly* 39 (1):49–72.

Stone, K. F., and H. Q. Dillehunt. 1973. *Self science: The subject is me*. Santa Monica: Goodyear Publishing Company.

Strasburger, L., Gutheil, T., and A. Brodsky. 1997. On wearing two hats: Role conflict in serving as both psychotherapist and expert witness. *American Journal of Psychiatry* 154:448–56.

Strupp, H. H. 1986. The nonspecific hypothesis of therapeutic effectiveness: A current assessment. *American Journal of Orthopsychiatry* 56 (4):513–20.

Styron, W. 1990. *Darkness visible*. New York: Random House.

Sutherland, A. 1996. Integrity and self-identity. *Philosophy* 35, supplementary volume:19–27.

Swanton, C. 2007. Virtue ethics, role ethics and business ethics. In *Working Virtues: Virtue Ethics and Contemporary Moral Problems,* ed. R. Walker and P Ivanhoe, 207–24. New York/Oxford: Oxford University Press.

Szabados, B., and E. Soifer. 2004. *Hypocrisy: Ethical investigations*. Peterborough: Broadview Press.

Szasz, T. 1974. *The myth of mental illness, revised edition*. New York: Harper Collins.

Taylor, C. 1989. *Sources of the self: The making of modern identity*. Cambridge, MA: Harvard University Press.

Taylor, C. 1992. Multiculturalism and the politics of recognition. In *Multiculturalism: Examining the politics of recognition*, ed. A. Gutmann, 25–74. Princeton: Princeton University Press.

Thomas, P. 1997. *The dialectics of schizophrenia*. London: Free Association Books.

Thompson, D. F. 2005. *Restoring responsibility: Ethics in government, business, and healthcare*. Cambridge: Cambridge University Press.

Tjeltveit, A. C. 1999. *Ethics and Values in Psychotherapy*. London: Routledge.

Tiberius, V. 2002. Perspective: A prudential virtue. *American Philosophical Quarterly* 39 (4):305–24.

Tong,. R. 1988. Towards an ethics for policy experts. *Policy Studies Journal* 16 (3):411–652.

Tong R. 1997. Feminist perspectives on empathy as an epistemic skill and caring as a moral virtue. *Journal of Medical Humanities* 18 (3):153–68.

Tong, R. 1998. The ethics of care: A feminist virtue ethics of care for healthcare practitioners. *Journal of Medicine and Philosophy* 23 (2):131–52

Topor, A. 2001. Dissertation. Managing the contradictions: Recovery from severe mental disorder. *Stockholm Studies of Social Work, Volume 18.* Stockholm: Stockholm University Press.

Ussher, J. 1991. *Women's madness: Misogyny or mental illness?* Amherst: University of Massachusetts Press.

U. S. Surgeon General. 1999. *Mental health: A report of the surgeon general.* Rockville: U. S. Department of Health and Human Services, Substance Abuse and Mental Health Services Administration, Center for Mental Health Services, and National Institutes of Health, National Institute of Mental Health.

Van Hooft, S. 1996. Bioethics and caring. *Journal of Medical Ethics* 22:83–9.

Van Hooft, S. 2005. *Understanding virtue ethics.* Chesham: Acumen Press.

Vawter, M. P., Evans, S., Choudary, P., et al. 2004. Gender-specific gene expression in postmortem human brain: localization to sex chromosomes. *Neuropsychopharmacology* 29:373–78.

Veatch, R. M. 1988. The danger of virtue. *The Journal of Medicine and Philosophy* 13:445–46.

Veatch, R. M. 1991. *The patient–physician relation: The patient as partner, part 2.* Bloomington: Indiana University Press.

Veatch, R. M. 2003. Is there a common morality? *Kennedy Institute Journal of Ethics* 13 (2):189–92.

Vehaak. 1993. Analysis of referrals of mental health problems by general practitioners. *British Journal of General Practice* 43 (370): 203–8.Vetlesen, A. J. 1994. *Perception, empathy and judgment: An inquiry into the preconditions of moral performance.* University Park: Pennsylvania University Press.

Wager, T., Phan, L., Liberzon, I., and S. Taylor. 2003. Valence, gender and lateralization of functional brain anatomy in emotion: A meta-analysis of findings from neuroimaging. *Neuroimage* 19:513–31.

Wahl, O. 1999. *Telling is risky business: Mental health consumers confront stigma.* New Brunswick, NJ: Rutgers University Press.

Wakeman, S. 2002. Working with the center: Psychiatric rehabilitation with people who dissociate. *Psychiatric Rehabilitation Journal* 26(2):115–122.

Watson, G. 1990. On the primacy of character. In *Identity, character and morality,* ed. O. Flanagan, A. Rorty, 449–70. Cambridge: MIT Press.

Weil, K. 1992. *Androgyny and the denial of difference.* Charlottesville: University of Virginia Press.

Wenegrat, B. 1995. *Illness and power: Women's mental disorders and the battle between the sexes.* New York: New York University Press.

Wertheimer, A. 1996. *Exploitation.* Princeton: Princeton University Press.

Whitaker, R. 2002. *Mad in America.* Cambridge: Perseus Publishing.

Widiger, T. A., and R. L. Spitzer. 1991. Sex bias in the diagnosis of personality disorders: Conceptual and methodological issues. *Clinical Psychology Review* 11:1–22.

Williams, B. A. O. 1986. *Ethics and the limits of philosophy.* Cambridge: Harvard University Press.

Woodruff, P. 2001. *Reverence: Renewing a forgotten virtue.* Oxford: Oxford University Press.

Yearley, L. H. 1990. *Mencius and Aquinas: Theories of virtue and conceptions of courage.* New York: State University of New York Press.

Zalta, A. K., and P. K. Keel. 2006. Peer influence on bulimic symptoms in college students. *Journal of Abnormal Psychology* 115 (1):185–89.

Zoppi K., and R. M. Epstein. 2002. Is communication a skill? *Communication Technique Behavior* 34: 319–24.

Author Index

Subject Index

accountability, 16, 71

advocacy, 18n, 19

agents of the state, 43

AIDS, 28

altruism, 155

Annotations Especially Applicable to Psychiatry, 22–24, 26, 28–29, 31, 51

antipsychiatry, 57

arête, 67

authenticity
  habituation and, 170, 173
  learning virtues and, 152, 157
  as metavirtue, 9, 106–107
  as psychiatric virtue, 142–144, 149, 186
  as virtue modifier, 108–109

autonomous agent/person
  dignity and, 136
  empathy and, 119n
  patient as, 19–22, 25
  severe mental illness and, 35, 56

autonomous self, 21n

autonomy
  as based upon virtues, 68
  consumer model and, 20–21, 56
  as ethical principle, 11–14, 61, 114–115
  gender identity and, 88, 100
  gender tropes and, 94
  patient, 7, 24–26, 31
  psychiatric power and, 112
  psychiatric setting and, 33–34
  relationship to other character traits, 128
  views about mental illness and, 42

beneficence, 11–12, 25–26, 68, 71, 163

boundaries (in the therapeutic relationship)
  long-term care and, 41–42
  phronesis and, 148
  psychiatric features of, 24–29, 31

boundaries (*cont.*)
  unselfing and, 9, 106, 132–134
  vulnerability and, 7
boundary violations, 27, 132, 141
brain injuries, 37

capabilities
  communicative, 14, 37, 100, 114, 130
  consumer model and, 20–21
  decisional, 25
  empathy and, 119–124
  human, 44, 48
  imaginative, 10, 202
  rational, 21
  reasoning, 14, 108
  serious mental illness and, 34–37, 42,
    135
  subcapabilities, 107–108, 119, 123–125,
    129, 168, 201–202
  perceptual, 119
  virtues as, 144, 149, 168, 201–202
  Western values and, 44
caring, 52, 209, 162, 172, 197
cases (dramaturgical)
  Case 1: Molecules and Marital Politics,
    178–181
  Case 2: Possible Predator, 181–186
  Case 3: Death Threats, 186–190
  Case 4: The Gatekeeper, 190–194
  Case 5: Paying for Psychotherapy,
    194–198
character. *See* virtues
chronicity, 22, 30, 40–41, 193
civil commitment, 43, 78–79, 112, 161,
    164
commodity, 19, 146
communicative exchange, 40, 130–131
community psychiatry, 56–58
compartmentalization
  bureaucracy and, 140–142
  integrity and, 165

risk to virtue, 9, 108
role specificity and, 154–155, 160–161
self and, 129
compassion
  empathy, relation to, 117–122
  good character and, 62
  healing and, 170
  as inner states, 134
  managed care and, 139–141
  mental disorders and, 14
  as motive, 64–65
  as virtue, 71, 74, 105–108, 117–122
  other virtues and, 112, 117–122
confidentiality, 79, 105, 109–111
Confucianism, 63n, 172
consumer model of patienthood, 19–21,
    31, 56, 138
countertransference, 51, 185
courage
  action and, 143
  as patient virtue, 5n, 35
  self-knowledge and, 128
  as virtue, 62, 66–67

depression
  case examples of, 28, 40, 179–180,
    181–184, 194–196
  chronicity, 40–42
  decision-making capacity and, 42
  empathy and, 28
  influence on the self, 34–37
  as major mental disorder, 34, 91
  treatment and, 52
  women and, 90, 95
diagnosis
  as ethical issue in psychiatry, 23–24
  as gendered, 91–93
  holism and, 48–49
  in managed care, 196
  as practice skill, 77
  as social construction, 29–31

.